Roll to Save

Gaming Disease Response

How to Construct Wargames in Support of Public Health Professionals

There are over one hundred books currently authored, co-authored or edited by John Curry as part of the History of Wargaming Project.

King R. and Curry J. (ed) (2015) It Could Happen Tomorrow! Emergency Planning Exercises for the Health Service deserves a note. Although it lacks an analytical framework, it is one of very few published examples of actual exercises carried out in the UK health sector.

Paddy Griffith's Counter Insurgency Wargames (1980)

Modern Crises Scenarios for Matrix Wargames

Peter Perla's Art of Wargaming book, A Guide for professionals and hobbyists

Thomas Allen's War Games: Professional Wargaming 1945-1985

Donald Featherstone's Solo Wargaming

Donald Featherstone's Wargaming Campaigns

Stuart Asquith's Wargaming 18th Century Battles: Including Rules for Marlburian Warfare 1702-1714

Innovations in Wargaming Vol 1, Developments in Hobby and Professional Wargames

Army Wargames: Staff College Exercises 1870-1980

Contact! The Restricted Canadian Army Tactical Wargame (1980)

Dunn Kempf: The Tactical Wargame of the American Army (1977-1997)

Tacspiel, the American Army's War Game of the Vietnam War (1966)

The British Army War Game (1956)

The British Army Desert War Game (1978) MOD Wargaming Rules

Andrew Wilson's The Bomb and the Computer: The History of Professional Wargaming 1780- 1968

See The History of Wargaming Project at www.wargaming.co for other publications.

The Red Die

Gaming Disease Response

How to Construct Wargames in Support of Public Health Professionals

_____

ED McGrady Ph.D. and John Curry

Edited by Peter Perla

The History of Wargaming Project

2021

Image credits (all used under license):

Cover Images: ID 119693427 © Tartilastock | Dreamstime.com
Figure 2: Map © OpenStreetMap contributors
Figure 3: Map © OpenStreetMap contributors
Figure 5: County Map of Virginia: ID 78880348 © Christian Mueller-clausnitzer | Dreamstime.com

First Printing: 2021

ISBN 9798720844516

The History of Wargaming Project

www.wargaming.co

Contents

Acknowledgements

I would like to thank my technical reviewers, Dr. Thomas Hertzheim, MD, Dr. Tim Creamer MD, and CAPT (RET.) Juliana Sadovich PhD, RN U.S. Public Health Service. They provided great insights and information to help this text, though all mistakes are my own.

Peter Perla not only read this text and gave extensive edits he has also been a good friend for a long time. I would like to thank him for everything, for giving me a boost into game design, for his advice and mentorship, but mostly his friendship throughout the years.

Finally, I would be remiss if I did not thank John Curry. He is a good friend and a better publisher, thoughtful and patient. Especially patient. Just what you would want in a publishing house.

ED McGrady

Foreword

Disease. It's recently been on our minds far more than perhaps ever before. The Covid-19 pandemic turned the world upside down and exposed the serious weaknesses in the readiness of many governments to respond to disease outbreaks. I'm not knowledgeable about the workings of the UK system of public health, but I have had some limited contact with that of the USA. Several years ago, I had the privilege of working with my friend and colleague, Ed McGrady, Ph.D., the author of this current tome, on a series of games sponsored by the Department of Health and Human Services (HHS) to explore public-health emergency response. During that effort we had the even greater privilege and pleasure of working with one of the giants of public-health history, D.A. Henderson, one of the leaders in the eradication of smallpox. Ed went on to develop and carry out several other "serious games" focused on biomedical issues, including bioterrorism and public-health responses.

The failures and confusion in the Covid-19 response of U.S. government agencies at the national, state and local levels reflected a failure to internalize the insights of some of those earlier games, as well as larger and more timely efforts, including a major 2019 game titled Crimson Contagion. This latter game—played by federal, state and local medical experts, politicians and officials—was based on a storyline which envisioned an influenza pandemic stemming from China. It took place only months before the eerily similar outbreak of Covid-19. The game identified several issues related to uncertainties about which agencies had the authority to take critical response to an evolving pandemic. Sadly, many of those issues showed themselves in the subsequent Covid-19 response operations.

This book makes no claims to be able to ensure that such errors of judgment, insight and operations will not take place in the future. What it does do, however, is provide a set of game-design concepts and examples, which current and future practitioners and officials can use to help themselves explore the scientific, organizational and political intricacies of dealing with disease outbreaks, large and small.

Perhaps even more than other types of serious games (such as the more well-known wargames) games dealing with disease and biomedical responses of all kinds must integrate both the scientific and storytelling aspects of what might be called representational, simulation, or decision-making games. Such serious games are referred to by many such terms, as well as other words such as tabletop exercises (or merely tabletops), seminar games, matrix games, even BOGSATs—bunch of guys sitting around a table. The validity and value of the insights stemming from these games remains a subject of debate within the community of gamers and "operators"— those responsible for taking action to formulate and carry out policy in the real world, which the games can only represent synthetically. Is such synthetic experience a valid basis for real action?

To explore that question—I certainly don't propose to give a definitive answer to it—allow me to ask another. What makes a human experience valid as opposed to correct or accurate? In a logical sense, may I draw valid conclusions from my own experience only to learn that those conclusions prove inaccurate when I confront a new set of circumstances different from the precise circumstances from which I drew my conclusions? Does that make my previous experience invalid? Or merely inapplicable? For example, I had a lot of experience driving a car in bad weather in Pittsburgh, where I grew up. When I tried to apply that experience to what seemed to be similar conditions in the Washington D.C. area, I was surprised to discover than the snow-covered roads in D.C. often concealed more icy conditions than I had experienced in Pittsburgh. My surprise was heightened by ending up in the median on U.S. Route 50 after a light tap of my brakes in slow traffic.

All of us, including public-health and government officials, have drawn certain conclusions based on our own experiences. To each, those experiences seem perfectly valid and applicable to their fields of responsibility and expertise. But because those experiences differ, so too do their interpretations of new and possibly unusual circumstances and their conclusions about how best to act. As we saw with Covid-19, there can be a high societal cost of waiting until an actual biomedical crisis to argue about what course of action might be more correct than others. So, what do we do?

It seems to me, then, that we must attempt to understand better what the various experts and decision makers think they have learned from their own experiences, what they presume each other have learned from theirs, and where might reside the objective reality of competing views. The types of biomedical gaming Dr. McGrady describes in this book can give us important tools for doing this because many of the most important issues we must confront are more about how people think, not merely how systems work. We must understand not only what they believe but also why they believe it. Why, for example, did so many in the general population prove so reluctant to get vaccinated against Covid-19?

Science tries to predict physical events and effects and calculate the chances that those predictions are correct. Science and clinical trials can estimate the efficacy of the various vaccines, but they cannot always calculate the answers to the human questions of beliefs and subsequent behaviors. Games can explore those answers and help us understand what we need to learn, or think, or guess to predict those answers. Can we do more?

Scientists who sometimes dismiss insights from games because of for their supposed lack of rigor and so lack of validity are arguing from the perspective of internal, or process, validity. If you cannot show the correctness of equations connecting the cause and outcome of a game writ large, then the game cannot be valid. But it that we're always true, no leap of creative insight that goes beyond the strict limits of standard logic would ever be valid. Yet, all real science depends on, indeed is driven by, precisely such creative leaps to point the way to new theories to be tested in new ways. What matters most in the real world is product, or external, validity; does the insight, regardless of how I got it, lead to behaviors or predictions that the real-world shows are correct or appropriate? It is here that serious games in general—and the games and design techniques described here in particular— find their true value. Games do not predict—people do. And will. And the insights produced by such biomedical games will factor into those human predictions, for good or ill. It requires the gaming, biomedical, political and bureaucratic communities to understand this fact, and together to improve our ability to design, run, and interpret disease-response games fairly and accurately if we are to avoid the ill and harvest the good.

This book is a roadmap pointing in the right direction…

Peter Perla

Washington, USA

February 2021

Chapter 1: Introduction

This book is about developing games in support of disease response operations. Both game design and disease response are broad and diverse topics. We will focus on game design through the lens of disease response. This means that we are not writing a book on designing professional games: there are other books for that.[1] Nor are we writing a book on disease, emergency response, or epidemiology: there are other books for that.[2]

And it's important to note that we are game designers and scientists who have done a lot of games working with the public health and medical communities. We are neither licensed doctors nor professional public health personnel. For medical advice please seek out a licensed medical professional. For public health emergencies find your local public health agency. And listen to them.

How do we build games that will affect and inform decision-making about disease response?

Well, we will need to draw from the medical and epidemiological literature in order to understand how diseases behave. We will need a detailed presentation of symptoms if medical personnel play. Some scenarios may require a worldwide projection of the evolution of a disease. Still other games may require an engineering study of how disease behaves in different environments. In some cases, we will need to do the basic epidemiology, especially in pandemic games or games that proceed to widespread community transmission.

We will need to build into our games the complex organizational, political, and governmental dynamics that define large-scale disease response operations. Looking at past disease response operations like the 2001 anthrax attacks,[3] the Zika event of 2017,[4] or the current COVID-19 response[5] we see that organizational and leadership decisions matter. That is often the most overlooked, and essential, part of disease response game design.

When we think of disease response, we think of the COVID-19 pandemic response of November 2019 through the foreseeable future.[6] But that is only one aspect of disease-response operations. Disease response is an ongoing and continuous problem for public health organizations. In 2020 the CDC had at least two major disease responses that required activation of its operations center. First was the response to vaping, and then COVID-19. Before that came the Ebola, Zika, and West Nile Virus disease response operations along with support to hurricane relief operations.[7] Those are very different response operations requiring different types of planning and coordination.

In addition to pandemics and "routine" activations, the disease response system also practices for intentional (and unintentional) release of biological agents. A lot of gaming on disease response outside of pandemics has involved games concerning the deliberate release of biological agents through terrorism. This, of course, has its own system and processes for response, different than either "routine" response or response to pandemics.

We can also characterize disease response operations according to the scale and scope of the effort. A case of food poisoning at a local salad bar[8] may generate what is an emergency response for a local health department, but that is a long way from the kind of international coordination required for a global pandemic. The different

---

[1] Perla, Peter with John Curry (ed.). (2012) Peter Perla's *The Art of Wargaming, 2nd Ed.*; Caffrey, Matthew. (2019) *On Wargaming.* Newport Papers 43. https://digital-commons.usnwc.edu/newport-papers/43/; Burns S. (ed.) (undated) Wargamer's Handbook. https://usnwc.edu/Research-and-Wargaming/Wargaming/Publications-and-Journals

[2] Timbrell, John A. (2009). *Principles of Biochemical Toxicology, 4th Ed.*; Steward, Antony. (2002) *Basic Statistics and Epidemiology;* Celentano, David and Moyses Szklo. (2019) *Gordis Epidemiology, 6th Ed.*; Johns Hopkins University, Red Cross, and Red Crescent. (2007) *Public Health Guide in Emergencies 2nd Ed.*

[3] Gursky, Elin, Thomas Inglesby, and Tara O'Toole. (2003) "Anthrax 2001: Observations on the medical and public health response." *Biosecurity and Bioterrorism: Biodefense Strategy, Practice, and Science.* 1:2.

[4] McNeil, Donald. (16 Jan 2017) "How the Zika response failed millions," *New York Times*

[5] Reuters (22 Apr 2020). "Special Report: Former Labradoodle Breeder Tapped to Lead U.S. Pandemic Task Force." *New York Times*

[6] This book is being written in the summer and fall of 2020. There is a large amount of uncertainty regarding how the SARS COVID-19 pandemic will play out, and this book studiously avoids any speculation on that point. For COVID-19 the time for games has pretty much passed. Though we will use a game on pandemic consequence management as an example later in the book, we are not focused on pandemics, or COVID-19, in this book.

[7] Centers for Disease Control and Prevention. https://emergency.cdc.gov/recentincidents/ accessed May 2020.

[8] See, for example, Torok, Thomas, et al. (6 Aug 1997) "A Large Community Outbreak of Salmonellosis Caused by Intentional Contamination of Restaurant Salad Bars," *Journal of the American Medical Association.* 278:5

scales of response will require different types of games, and different gaming techniques. They each have their own set of challenges, decisions, and opportunities for the game designer.

In this book we do not plan to favor any particular route for the emergence of a disease response. We will cover disease and disease response in general, and then discuss the specific elements of response to intentional, pandemic, or routine disease spread. We will also discuss different scale games, from a game that looks at distribution of prophylaxis and vaccine at an individual site to a multi-national game involving an international pandemic.

Given the ongoing (as we write) outbreak of COVID-19/novel coronavirus-19 this book takes on a serious and solemn dimension. Games were put on before the outbreak and informed many of the experts' ruminations on whether and how to respond to COVID-19.[9] However, the results show us the sobering news that no matter how accurate, predictive, or engaging our games are, decision-makers will often ignore the insights they produce.[10] Political leaders have many different things to balance, and hypotheticals are pretty low on most priority lists.[11]

That should not stop us from developing games on disease response. It should make us even more aware of the responsibility that we have in developing those games. Responsibly to get the science right, or as right as we can. To be skeptical of easy numbers and estimates. Responsibility to make sure that we include the political, social, and individual rivalries and bad behaviors in our games. And to communicate the results clearly, effectively, and to the right people. It is literally the best we can do. The rest is up to the decision-makers.

So why should this book matter to you?

If you are a health care systems analyst you may find yourself involved in either game construction, or participation in games. Often these games are not designed by people familiar with the field, or the designers focus on the agent[12] not the players. Either way it may be useful for you to understand the game where you are a participant.

If you are an operations analyst, you may be asked to observe a game and build a model based on the game results. Ignoring whether or not that is a good idea,[13] you may benefit from understanding what should be going on in the game, and how the designers likely came to their design.

Finally, if you are a game designer who has been asked to build a game on disease response, this book may give you a starting point for choosing your agent, shaping your scenario, and engaging the players. It may help dissuade you from using an over-the-top model that makes it look like everyone is going to die and the situation is hopeless. It usually isn't, and that gives everyone the wrong impression of the problem. Professional games are about getting the players to think about events in new and creative ways, ways that they will need to think during an actual event. Because actual events are unpredictable, messy, and require that plans be adapted and changed.

Which brings us to the question of the role of epidemiology in building games on disease response. Or, for that matter, medical information in general. Games are not pretending to be predictive the way some modeling is, so let's understand up front that adding a game wrap-around to a model will not make either one more predictive. In the COVID-19 event, models, data, and understanding are all ever changing and quite diverse depending on who you talk to.

Will we do epidemiological modeling in this book?

No. Neither of us are MD/M.Ph.'s and we do not have their level of expertise in modeling or tracking down a disease. We won't pretend like we do. Our games will use epidemiological models, since its critical to 'get it

---

[9] Sanger, David, et al. (22 Mar 2020) "Before the Outbreak a cascade of warnings went unheeded." *New York Times*.. https://nyti.ms/2U1tyAs

[10] Ellis, Devin. (2020) "'Crimson Contagion' – What can we learn?" *PAXSims Blog.* https://paxsims.wordpress.com/2020/03/19/crimson-contagion-what-can-we-learn/

[11] Political leaders always have to balance between the demands of what is happening right now, with the expense and difficulty of preparing for what might be. It can be difficult for political leaders to spend resources on something that might happen, but no one has experienced yet. The idea of planetary defense became a bigger issue after the Shoemaker-Levy 9 comet impacted Jupiter, simply because everyone had seen it happen. See, for example, https://www.nasa.gov/feature/goddard/2019/how-historic-jupiter-comet-impact-led-to-planetary-defense

[12] E.g. the virus

[13] Games use models as we will see in later chapters. However, models and games are fundamentally different ways of understanding problems, and should not be conflated.

right' when building a game. We will discuss the practical elements of modelling, and how to use them in our games.

Our perspective on models, and any other data, is a practical one. We want to build the most accurate and compelling game possible, without becoming modelers ourselves.

We will start off by building an understanding of both game design and disease response. While this is not a book is not solely focused on designing games, we do have to build a baseline understanding of what is involved in game design before we can proceed. We also need to build a baseline understanding of what elements of medicine, biology, and epidemiology are needed for the game designer. Then we will proceed to associate game design and biology through the process of building strategic, operational, and tactical disease-response games. After that we will move into some special topics, such as matrix games (a particular kind of narrative role-playing game), that always seem to be on everyone's mind.

Throughout this book we will give example game problems and game designs in response. These are designed to illustrate the points we make in the text, but also give us the chance to give practical tips and advice on game design and execution. The examples reflect real life but are not associated with real-world events.

As always, our goal in this book will be to outline the art of games design as applied to disease response operations in order to help professionals to better prepare for the next crisis.

Chapter 2: What are games?

The best answer to the question "what are games?" is "games are hard to define!" In this chapter we will discuss this problem a bit more, say why it's extremely important for you to understand and then attempt to describe what we mean when we talk about games.

The Definition Problem

Whenever I teach about games I always start with this quote from Wittgenstein:[14]

> 66. Consider for example the proceedings that we call "games". I mean boardgames, card-games, ball-games, Olympic games, and so on. What is common to them all? --- Don't say "There must be something common, or they would not be called 'games' " --- but look and see whether there is anything common to all. --- For if you look at them you will not see something that is common to all, but similarities, relationships, and a whole series of them at that. To repeat: don't think, but look! --- Look for example at board-games with their multifarious relationships. Now pass to card-games; here you may find many correspondences with the first group, but many common features drop out, and others appear..... And we can go through the many, many other groups of games in the same way; can see how similarities crop up and disappear. And the result of this examination is: we see a complicated network of similarities overlapping and criss-crossing: sometimes overall similarities, sometimes similarities of detail.

> 67. I can think of no better expression to characterize these similarities than "family resemblances"; for the various resemblances between members of a family: build, features, colour of eyes, gait, temperament, etc. etc. overlap and criss-cross in the same way. --- and I shall say: 'games' form a family. – Wittgenstein[15]

What I take away from this quote is that "game" is a term that means many things to different people. It depends both on context, as well as the experience of the users. If you say, "it's this thing" then someone else can come along and say, "but what about this?" The similarities and differences between all of the objects that fall under the rubric of "game" form a family of relationships, a network of meanings and associations, that give us a sense that we "know" what we are talking about when we use the term, but we really don't have an independent, objective, definition because there is no shared meaning.

This matters a lot for the game designer. It is one of the fundamental problems that we face. There are two aspects to this problem: communications and inheritance.

Communications: When we communicate about games, with sponsors, players, or those not involved in the game, we need to understand that we are using a language that is both imprecise and subject to misinterpretation. What we mean by "game" may not be what my sponsor or player means by the term. Those internal definitions are shaped by personal experience and analysis, and they may not be the same.

This means that as designers we have to be careful with our language when we talk about games. Too often we know what we mean but our listeners won't have any idea what we mean. Or, worse, they will be thinking of something else. We can get around this by carefully describing the meaning of our terms. How, exactly, will players participate in our games? What will the game entail? How might our game be different from others that the player may have experienced? Grounding our definitions in practical terms is always the best way to ensure common understanding.

The challenge is that mis-understanding will lead to crossed intentions, poorly executed design, and hurt feelings. No one wants that.

Inheritance: The challenge of inheritance extends the above challenge to all of the different terms we use for games. Serious games, professional games, wargames, tabletops, exercises, simulations, seminar games, and role-playing games all will inherit the definitional challenge from the root term "game." This means we also have a challenge in defining what we mean by different types of games.

---

[14] ED McGrady
[15] Wittgenstein, Ludwig. (1958) *Philosophical Investigations*.

You would think this might be a bit easier, because different types of games are generally specific in their style and execution than generic "games." However, there is no standard set of definitions for different types of games, despite efforts to define them.[16] That means when I say "tabletop game" I may mean a game with a map on a table, a discussion, or a game held sitting around a table. Likewise, for the ubiquitous "seminar" and "matrix" games. There are things that we, and many other designers, think about when we use those terms, but there are also a large number of things that other people may also think about.

Again, detailed description of what exactly is intended will save the game designer from any misunderstandings which could lead to later irritation and disappointment (or shock and surprise).

Defining Games

There are many definitions of "game" or "wargame." My definitions, derived from many conversations with Peter Perla and others, are:

> *Game*: people, making decisions, in a simulated environment, where they get to see the consequences of those decisions.

> *Wargame*: people, making decisions, in a simulated conflict environment, where they get to see the consequences of those decisions.

These definitions emphasize what is important in games: they are about people, who make decisions with consequences.

For other examples of the definition of "game" and "wargame" see, for example, Caffrey (2019).[17]

One way to divide games is by intent or purpose. Games for entertainment have very different criteria for design success than do games that will be played by professionals. In this book we will be focused on these "professional games."[18]

Of course, this leaves out games for spiritual or religious purposes,[19] gambling, educational, or serious games. The serious games movement may object, saying that serious games fall into the professional category. However, while serious games can be professional games, they also can be used to entertain or inform patients in the hospital or other places. They can also be used to educate. They fall into a gray area that includes several different game objectives.

Even the simple distinction, between professional and serious games, is fraught with definitional and categorical problems. It is a perfect example of what I mean by the inheritance of Wittgenstein's point about the term "game."

Professional games, by my definition, are games played by professionals for purposes other than entertainment. It is not that the games they play should not be entertaining, it's just that is not their primary purpose.

We also need to take a moment and describe what games are not.

- *Games are not puzzles*, though games often incorporate puzzles. Puzzles are often called games, think of the digital game *Myst* as an example. Puzzles are one of those definitional gray areas, but professional games are not puzzles.

- *Meetings are not games.* The difference between a game and a meeting is that something *happens* in a game. Games move through time. The situation in the game evolves, and it evolves based on choices that the players make. A meeting begins and ends by discussing the set of points or topics that was the subject of the meeting. It proceeds linearly through real time, and it has no "game time" or time that is

---

[16] Simpson, William. Ed. (20 Sept 2017) *A Compendium of Wargaming Terms* . https://usnwc.edu/Research-and-Wargaming/Wargaming/Publications-and-Journals

[17] The section The Taxonomy of Wargaming in Caffrey (2019) p. 261 has a list of various definitions.

[18] This is my preferred term for what we are doing as it conveys both professionalism as well as the target audience for the game. It has less ambiguity than terms like "serious game," wargame, "analytic game" or any number of other terms that are often used.

[19] Which, surprisingly, is a thing, and indeed a very old thing. Roberts, John, et al. (1959) Games *in Culture*. American Anthropologist. 61

independent of real time. Likewise, the participants don't get to see the consequences of their action, unless the action occurs in the real world.

- *Professional games are not hobby games.* Hobby games, or generally games for entertainment, are often confused with professional games, or they are considered as possible substitutes. For a whole host of reasons, it is very difficult to simply substitute an off-the-shelf game for a professional game without extensive reworking. Most professional games need to be designed specifically for the application involved because professionals require detail, and accuracy in things like organizational relationships, that are often overlooked by hobby designers[20].

- *Games are not gamification.* Gamification is another term that is used loosely and can be used to refer to professional games. That is incorrect. Gamification is a whole discipline in itself. Essentially gamification seeks to use game-like incentives and mechanics to shape behavior. It is more complex and subtle than that, but it does not involve the same objectives or mechanics that professional games do.

- *Games are not game theory.* Game theory is yet another term that is confused with gaming. Game theory is a subset of mathematical economics that seeks to understand trade-offs in conflict and choice. Other than the use of the term "game" game theory has no relationship to what we are talking about. Though, sometimes, game theory can be used to analyze particular challenges that are set up in games. But that is an analysis, not a game design, tool.

- *Games are also not exercises.* Exercises, as discussed in Peter Perla's book (Perla, 2012), involve taking forces out into the field and seeing if they can execute an operation. This is an important component of Perla's "cycle of research" which involves games identifying the concepts, analysis providing quantitative assessment, and exercises providing a practical assessment of the concepts. In a game you can think of many things that you might do with your forces, but once you get real people with real equipment in the field you may find it harder to execute those ideas than you thought. That is what exercises do, they test concepts against reality. With real people and equipment.

Finally, *games are neither models nor simulations.* Models seek to represent a physical process or part of nature. Simulations bring multiple models together into an integrated process. Games can use models and simulations, but they are neither models nor simulations. They focus on people, the decisions they make and the changes that happen when people actively confront each other. Games might be thought of as a simulation that runs on the minds of the players.[21]

Below the top-level definitions, professional games are a very diverse group of games. For the purposes of this book, we can focus on the basic types of professional games. These are shown in table 1

Professional games	
Purpose	Mechanics
Training	Discussion
Education	Seminar
Understanding	Scenario
Exploration	Map-based
Organizational	Role-playing
Business	Matrix
	Computer moderated
	Virtual/Augmented reality

Table 1: Types of professional games

In the table above you see we have all of the same problems we discussed previously. You can have a seminar game that involves a map and role playing. You can have a map-based game that is facilitated like a seminar.

---

[20] Not necessarily as the hobby designers are unaware, but they make design decisions about the focus for their games reflecting the interest of their target audience.

[21] Sometimes as a game designer you will be required to refer to your product as a "simulation" simply because no one will participate in, or fund, a game. The word simulation sounds much fancier and more scientific, so you kind of have to go with it. I like to think that we are using a broader meaning of "simulation" to mean a small representation of reality as opposed to a gigantic computer program.

I also contend educational and training games are professional games, even though they also fall into the serious games category. So, already, the definitions are becoming fluid and complex.

In addition to the above categories of game, games can be divided up according to how they are controlled, and how information flows in the game.

Games control can be characterized as *rigid* or *free*. Rigid games have a formal set of rules which the players or controllers execute. Board games like chess are the most common example of rigid games. In chess players are responsible for executing the game based on the rules. The rules tell the players everything you need to know about the game, from how to set it up, to how to win.

Free games involve a controller assisting the players in executing the game. In free games some or all of the rules are created during the game. The rules are based on the current circumstances and the understanding of the controller. The most common example of a free game is the role-playing game *Dungeons and Dragons*. In most role-playing games there is a *dungeon master* responsible for running the game and managing the players actions. While the dungeon master has fixed rules they can refer to, they can also deviate from the rules when they need to, or create new rules based on the situation.

Free *Kriegsspiel* (for the German term for "wargaming") as it is called is a very common format for professional games. There may be fixed rules, but it is up to the controller to walk the players through the rules and use their expert judgment when they do or don't apply. In our experience there is little tolerance amongst professional players for sitting down and learning a complex set of rules, then playing a rigid game by them. They have better things to do (like fighting disease).

We can also group games according to how they deal with information. *Open games* provide the players with all, or most, of the information available in the game. Chess is an open game where each player knows the location and type of their own and the other player's units. Both players also know the rules and objectives of the game.

In a *closed game* some of the information in the game is hidden from the players. Common examples are the location or strength of enemy units, as in *Stratego*, or the other player's victory conditions as in many Eurogames.[22] The nature, amount, and methods of hiding information can vary greatly from game to game.

Most games designed for disease response follow the general format of other professional games. They combine some rigid elements, such as disease progression, with mostly free adjudication and control of player actions. They are also mostly open games, with players knowing what is going on within their scope of work. However, some information, such as the progression of the disease, the index cases, or other information may be withheld from the players until certain actions have occurred or a certain amount of game time has expired.

How Games are Organized

While games come in all shapes and sizes they are made up of some basic elements. These will be discussed in greater detail later, but a brief outline is included below.

Most professional games will have a *sponsor*. The sponsor determines the games *objectives* and works with the designer to achieve those objectives under various *constraints* that are imposed on the game. The game designer takes the objective and their own knowledge of games and builds a game design that includes everything from how the game will be played, or *mechanics*, to the appearance and presentation of the game *materials*. Throughout the design process the designer is doing *analysis* to understand the problem and identify the best way to construct the game *scenario* and other elements.

When the game happens *players* will make decisions and a *controller* will help guide them through the game and *adjudicate* the outcomes of their decisions. The controller is the person in overall charge of how the game runs, and they determine what everyone else in the game other than the players is doing. Often controllers will

---

[22] Eurogames are hobby games that emphasize abstract mechanics and indirect player interaction. They also tend to have multiple paths to victory and a more economic, rather than combat, emphasis. This includes mechanics like auctions, worker placement, or trading and negotiation. *Settlers of Catan, Agricola*, and *Ticket to Ride* are all examples of popular Eurogames. The innovative mechanics and complex paths to victory in these games have made them hugely influential on all forms of modern gaming. The games' lack of conflict and avoidance of military themes made them initially popular in Europe, especially Germany, and hence the term "Eurogames."

input events into the game, or *injects*, that will give the players additional information, represent follow-on events, or respond to player actions.

Colors are often used in games to designate different groups. In the United States control is referred to as the "white" cell, the players are divided into the good actors – the blue cell, and the not so good actors or the red cell. Non-aligned actors would be the green cell. Many other colors can be used but these are the standard ones.

The game runs through a series of *turns* or *moves* for a pre-determined length of time. At the end of the game there is often a *"hot wash"* or debrief, where players discuss their actions, and review the overall course and design of the game. After some time, a report is usually issued that covers what happened in the game and any insights derived from play.

This terminology throughout the book when referring to games and game components.

Chapter 3: Tactical Vaccine/Prophylaxis Game

The best way to understand what a professional disease response game looks like is to describe one. Let us start at the most basic level, with a game designed to help a local county health department distribute treatments or prophylaxis. This is a common problem in U.S. homeland security gaming. Distributing medical treatments or prophylaxis can occur as part of almost any widespread disease response operation, and it involves considerable coordination and a remarkable number of decisions.

In order to make these examples more concrete we will be using the State of Florida as a location for our scenarios. In particular we will focus on Brevard County, Florida which is an ideal representation of a small to medium sized county with a diverse set of industries, including tourism, as well as national security with the Kennedy Space Complex located at its northern end and the Harris Corporation located at its southern end.[23] Figure 1 shows the outline of the county.

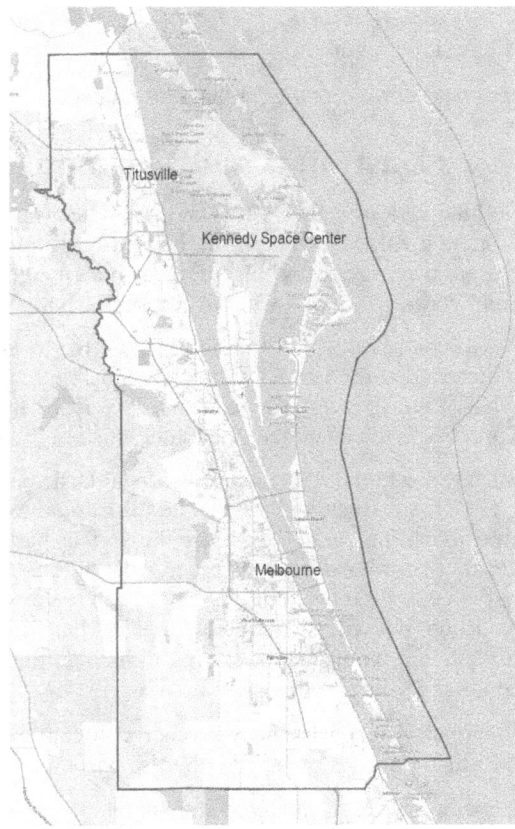

Figure 1 – Brevard County, Florida

Note that our games and scenarios are not based on official scenarios, intelligence, or frankly any insights other than we like this area of Florida and are familiar with it. Our descriptions, particularly of process or government structure may be significantly different than those in the areas discussed. It is likely any real-world response will be different from our descriptions. It would not be advisable to use this simplified response for the purposes of the game in the real world. It is simply an example of game design considerations.

To be clear, this is all made up. Fictional. Not real. If you want real information about these topics talk to the officials from the organizations involved. And do visit the space and treasure coasts as a tourist, they are quite lovely.

---

[23] This specificity will also allow us to reference homeland security plans, which are widely available on the web. For Florida public health exercises see: http://www.floridahealth.gov/programs-and-services/emergency-preparedness-and-response/training-exercise/exercise.html

Game Objectives

During a public health response various types of medicinal may need to be distributed to the public. This can range from vaccines to antibiotics to other forms of prophylaxis or treatment. To do this the supplier will typically send a bulk shipment of material, which then needs to be broken down, transported to the distribution site, and distributed. Given the often-fraught nature of the situation security may be needed, and careful organization and planning are required. Clear and precise public communications are also required so that the population understands what it should do, and why. One way governments explore the planning process is through a game designed to bring everyone together and figure out who is going to do what when. The problem is so complex it is difficult to comprehend, but the format of a game can help visualize this situation and highlight key issues.[24]

The county health department wants to understand:

- What will be required of various organizations and groups (police, emergency services, public health, local government, etc.) during the distribution of essential medicinals during a major public health response.

- How the distribution site will be set up.

- What coordination needs to occur with other organizations, especially the federal and state levels.

Constraints and Assumptions

The game will need to include all the various stakeholders and, we will assume for this game, can only last one day. Since many of the stakeholders involved will be from the first-response community, who are accustomed to action, we will want to make sure there are many different ways to engage with the game. People learn and interact with the world in different ways, so we will want to combine talking with the players doing something.

The plan for dispersal already exists and will need to be made available to us from the Florida Department of Health (FDOH).[25] This plan indicates that the FDOH will be responsible for receiving materials from the U.S. Strategic National Stockpile (SNS)[26] at a Receipt, Stage, and Store (RSS) facility. We can assume that other providers will follow a similar process in the event that the material is not drawn from the SNS.

From this facility FDOH will push the material to the county's Local Distribution Site (LDS) which in turn will be sent to Point of Dispensing (POD) sites where they will be distributed to the population. We will need to account for all of this in the game, assuming we will even use the SNS as part of the game. Not using SNS will require players from the state to figure out how they will receive the bulk material and how they will distribute it. There is also the challenge of what to do if you don't have enough material to meet the local demands. The FDOH has a Medical Advisory Group that will determine who gets what/when if supplies fall short. If FDOH is a major participant in the game then it would be interesting to include this as part of the process and let the county "compete" with other counties for its place in the line to receive timely supplies.

There are legal issues associated with having the authority to receive stockpile materials, who directs distribution, and who is in charge. So, we will likely need some legal expertise participating in the game.

You can have issues with some medicinals requiring cold storage or special handling, resulting in requirements for refrigeration in storage and transport.

There has been considerable planning, and prior gaming, of this problem. Because of this, we will need access to subject matter experts in the FDOH and emergency management community that can walk us through both the process, and the issues that remain, so that we can structure the game as realistically as possible. It is well

---

[24] The strength of the game is the highlight key issues that would have been unlikely to have emerged just from a discussion.

[25] Florida Department of Health (FDOH). (27 Jan 2015) *Strategic National Stockpile Standard Operating Procedure.* Ver. 1.4.

[26] The United States Department of Health and Human Services has multiple stockpiles of different types of medicines and treatments staged in warehouses ready to be deployed during an event. In the latest COVID-19 event the stockpile ventilators were referenced as a resource that could be sent to the states. These assets can be deployed quickly and are designed to be distributed within hours of activation. In some cases, such as doxycycline distribution in response to an anthrax attack, this is required by the nature of the event and agent involved.

known that the act of designing such a game is a method to developing understanding of the situation being modelled.

The Players

The players in a game like this will probably arrive somewhat cynical because they have participated in a lot of tabletop exercises, and are well versed in their emergency response plans. They have rehearsed, learned, and are intimately familiar with their plans and authorities and will be very sensitive to any deviation from the plan. No one will want to look bad. So, we are going to have a lot of fun putting in a scenario they had neither planned for, nor thought through, before.[27]

Key players would include:
- State of Florida Department of Health
- Brevard County Department of Health
- Brevard County Hospital System (both the association and individual hospitals)
- State Department of Law Enforcement
- Local law enforcement
- Local leadership (county supervisor or mayors)

Other possible players, depending on the sensitivity of the situation could include:
- Players representing the general public
- Legal representatives to advise at the state, local, and public interest level
- Media
- Local businesses, especially those dealing with national security
- Local military base representatives (not health)

Since most of these players would be from the organization and agency represented in the game, no additional training or information about the roles would be needed. Even people playing the general public would not need a lot of training, as they would indeed be part of the general public in their real lives. If the players did not have experience in their roles then they would either need a short training session, or cards and materials describing their roles.

This is a small, tactical level, game that is typical for rehearsing and preparing for medical response to homeland security events. It is different from most of these events in that it has the players planning, and then seeing the outcome of those plans. The inclusion of queuing models or other ways to simulate the actual distribution process would further distinguish this game from the majority of distribution games.

Game concept

The good news is that we can avoid a lot of the challenges associated with pre-planning and all of the processes and procedures that the players will know by heart by simply going off script and not using the SNS. Let's assume it is a vaccine, one that requires cold storage, which needs to be distributed. The vaccine is population specific; the younger cohorts are more vulnerable to the virus and thus anyone under 30 will receive the first round of vaccinations. (This should complicate things in Florida.). In addition, to make distribution more complicated, national security workers will also be eligible for the vaccine according to federal guidance.

By changing up the system this will allow us to test the concept and intent of the distribution plan, without having the players robotically work through something they have worked thorough several times before.

The Florida aliquot of the vaccine will arrive at the State RSS facility located in Orlando Florida near the Orlando International Airport.[28] In turn the vaccine will be loaded, still in its original 300 dose boxes, into Florida

---

[27] This is an assumption; I have no real idea what they have or have not thought through. However, I do know that this type of response process gets thoroughly planned and extensively rehearsed.

[28] At this point the scenario becomes fictional, we have no idea where the Florida RSS is actually located or whether there is even warehouse and storage facilities of this type at the Orlando Airport. In a real design we would be relying on state and local experts to guide us in what would make sense and comply with security requirements.

National Guard refrigerated trucks[29] where it will be escorted by the Florida State Police and Florida National Guard to Brevard's LDS. A National Guard contingent from Brevard will receive the vaccines and then it is up to the local Department of Health to take it from there.

Since the distribution will be to less than the whole population, and we are assuming a virus that will be a threat to the whole population but primarily those under the age of 30, there will need to be security for the vaccine throughout the distribution process. There may also need to be crowd and traffic control at the site. Not everyone will speak English, and informed consent will have to be obtained from all who are vaccinated. This includes counseling on side-effects, questions about allergies, etc. In addition, the county will have to figure out a way to get the affected population to the sites, whether they can vaccinate everyone from that population on the first round, and how to distinguish those who have been vaccinated from those who are not. There will be a lot of things for the county health department to figure out.

They will also need to lay out the physical site where people will be vaccinated. Now we could construct it so that they only lay out the inside of the building, or buildings, but it's likely that the area around the building will need a perimeter for security, and a further perimeter for traffic control. Given it's Florida there will be little or no public transportation so there will need to be extensive parking. Some will likely come by bus, so there will need to be accommodations for different sized vehicles. So, we will probably want a map and pieces representing all of the elements that could be positioned inside a Point of Distribution. We will also need queuing models or at least some way to give feedback to the participants about how their layout is working.

Figure 2 shows a sample layout for a small vaccination POD. In this case it is set up in a school auditorium and cafeteria. The patients enter and check-in, then proceed through counseling, vaccination, and recovery. We put security up on the stage so they could oversee the entire operation. Before using this in the game we will need to calculate throughput and understand how changes that players may make (adding stations, for example) will affect throughput. There may also be other steps that the players want to take, like distribution and management of protective equipment, rest areas for staff, and technology for registration and record keeping.

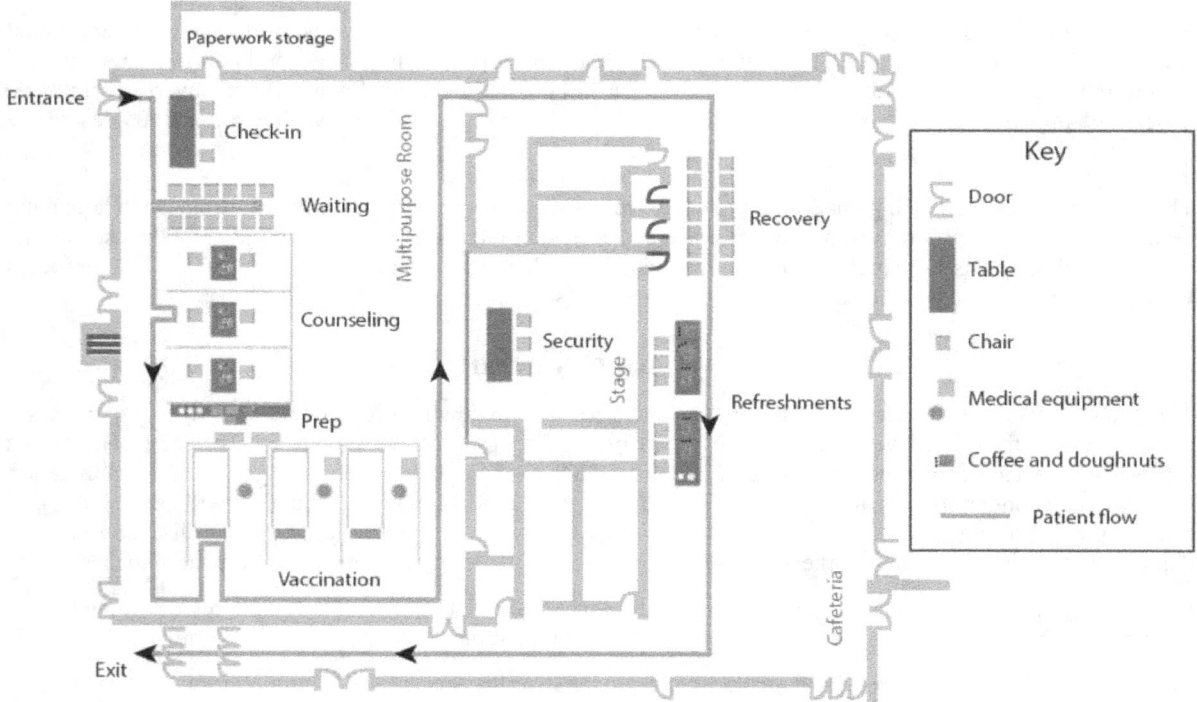

Figure 2 – Vaccine distribution POD sample layout

Game turns will be variable in length. We will want to emphasize planning and thinking, so there will be a long initial planning phase before the vaccine arrives. Once the vaccine arrives, we will hand it off to the county representatives and they will determine how long it takes between the various logistics wickets it goes through.

---

[29] Where, when, and how the Guard will get its refrigerated trucks, or when it will be told it needs them, will be part of game play.

Typically, these are receiving, inventory, breaking the supply down for further distribution (remember we kept the vaccine in the original packages? There was a reason we did that.), and movement to the POD, and then organizing for distribution.

After the distribution has begun game control will introduce the inevitable protests, security challenges, and disruptions that would occur at a POD. We may even include a lawsuit challenging the legality of the prioritization. We will end the game with a "hot washup." This refers to an out of role discussion of what was learned from the game, and what actions might be taken to better prepare for an actual event.

What seems like a simple game suddenly becomes a relatively complicated set of decisions. Its far more than "we get the stuff, and hand it out." Understanding the basics of that process and some of the issues that will occur is essential in designing the game. This can come from you own experience (which is what we are relying on here) or from subject matter experts (which is what we would rely on in a real design). But the game will be an opportunity to get the players to think outside of the standard plans and responses they have been trained to do. It will require them to synthesize information, work together, and make decisions in the game, so that when faced by crises in the real world they can make faster and better decisions. That is what games do.

Game execution

In this section we describe the first two turns of the game. We do this in order to give you an idea of how the game might be executed, along with some of the decisions and actions the game controller might take during the course of the game.

Pre-game

At the beginning of the game, we will assemble all of our players and go through a description of the game, the purpose of the game, and the scenario. We will want to end with the initial scenario situation so that the players can easily move right into the game. We will divide the players into three groups: the medical community including the hospitals and public health, the public safety community including any leadership like mayors or council members, and the security community to include the local police, sheriff, and FBI. Until a disaster is declared and an incident command system is stood up these entities would work the problem separately and from their own perspectives.

Turn 1

We would want to begin the game somewhat ahead of time prior to the arrival of the vaccine so that some planning could occur. Thus turn 1 is the "pre-arrival" turn where everyone needs to get ready to receive the vaccine. The vaccine has arrived at the State RSS facility and the State has sent liaison officers to work with Brevard County in formulating their plan. Key elements of the plan that the State expects from the County include:

- Who, exactly, will provide security and if it is the Brevard National Guard when and how will the activation request be issued from the County to the State Emergency Operations Center for approval by the Governor? There is a lead time for their mobilization and deployment.
- What role will local LEA have in managing the event? Will they require details from the local PD and/or Sherriff's office?
- Where will the vaccine be received, and what capabilities do they have for storage, breakdown, and packaging? Who will do all this since the County DOH is not overflowing with personnel.[30]
- Have the vaccination sites been identified and how will it be transported?
- What is the layout of the vaccination sites, where will the personnel come from, and how will vaccination proceed?
- What is the command and control laydown for the operation, who is communicating with who, who is in charge, and what decisions require higher authority authorization.

We will have developed a model that can incorporate transportation and distribution of the vaccine at the county level. It may be as straightforward as a spreadsheet or it could be as sophisticated as a complex simulation. We

---

[30] For game purposes we are making some assumptions here. This may, or may not, be the case but all of our assumptions are common ones.

will also have a simulation of the vaccination site ready to go that can be adapted to their plan. As they come up with options and designs control will be modifying or updating these systems so they are ready to go for turn 2.

At the end of this turn the vaccine will have arrived, and the distribution process begun.

Turn 2

Now that the distribution process to the vaccination sites has begun, we will want to understand how their plan compares with the reality and friction of operations. To do this we will have pre-scripted "injects" or events that will make their lives more difficult. In no way is this the end of the world, rather they are the standard kinds of hiccups that occur in situations like this. These will be given to the players at the beginning of the turn, and the players will have to work out solutions under the limits imposed by their previous decisions. Injects will be based on player decisions from Turn 1, but they might include:

- Loss of refrigeration at one or more sites.
- Media and social media complaints, and possibly protests and civil actions, by senior citizens demanding that the distribution of the vaccine be more "equitable and fair." This would be exacerbated by media reporting of deaths amongst the senior population.
- Sites that are crowded or jammed by those seeking vaccine.
- Corruption of the registration or other online/phone processes designed to manage appointments and space out the uptake of the vaccine. This could range from simple over subscription or access to web pages to delivery hacking to various fraudulent schemes.
- Demand for tracking and inventory of vaccines, with a constant "how's it going" drumbeat from the State and Federal officials.
- Local rumors and events regarding vaccine side effects such as allergic reactions or militant anti-vaxers.
- Local issues such as heat effects, humidity, and other conditions that could affect distribution. For example, Kennedy Space Center workers are suddenly declared essential and the federal government attempts to take vaccine supplies and sites for its own use.

These and other events will complicate the process of distribution for the County and require them to develop work-arounds, and test their command and control and planning processes.

Turn 3

Now we will move into the vaccine site, with players assuming roles within the context of one of their own vaccination delivery sites. We will include additional injects, many depending on actions from Turns 1 and 2. For example, if they refused to deal with anti-vaxers in Turn 2 they could show up at the site and be disruptive. Depending on site security this could be easily handled, police are called and individuals arrested, or more difficult, armed private security guards engage with the individuals, it goes badly and the site is disrupted.

By the end of Turn 3 most of those participating in the exercise will have had enough. And we can now turn to the hotwashup, where everyone gets to talk about what they learned, what they would do differently, and how plans, procedures, and expectations need to change in order for the event to be successful in the real world. For example, the County may not have any way to call on the National Guard, which would be noted from the game and a process and procedure put in place in consultation with the State Guard office and the County emergency management office.[31]

---

[31] Again, we are making things up for purposes of illustration. Brevard County may indeed have an excellent way of managing their interactions with the State Guard, they probably do because they do it so often for hurricanes.

Chapter 4: Designing Professional Games

This is not a book on how to design professional games in general. That is a subject in itself. However, it is a book on designing professional games for disease response, so we will cover the basics of professional game design.

A good game design challenges the players by using all of the game elements, from scenario to materials, to surprise and delight in the players and put them into the game world and give them a flow experience. Most of the rest of this chapter will be in explaining what that sentence means.

Elements of a Game

There are many ways to approach a discussion of game design, and there are many other books on game design.[32] I am going to start by describing the parts of a professional game. Table 2 shows the internal and external elements of a game.

Elements of a game	
Outer	Inner
Objective	Dramaturgical
Players	Gameplay
Scenario	Narrative
Mechanics	Neurological
Materials	Social
Venue	Frame
Constraints	Humanistic
Observation	

Table 2 – Elements of a game

We will focus on the "outer" elements of a game, and only briefly cover the inner elements.

Outer elements

Objectives

If you take any course on professional game design, or just ask any professional game designer, you will hear that objectives are the most important part of game design. Like the foundation for a house the whole project may fall down unless you have a good grounding on what you are trying to do.

While knowing what you are doing and why you want to do it is essential on taking on any project, from building a table and chairs to designing an airplane, it is critical in game design. A sponsor will ask for a game on a response to smallpox. That is a very broad and general topic. What, exactly, is the sponsor trying to understand? It will be a very different game if the sponsor wants to understand how their decisions will affect the timeline for the disease compared to a game where they want to examine the initial process of notifications and public communications.

There are several ways to get more specific on objectives. The Naval War College[33] in their wargame's handbook has the sponsor and designer both signing off on a design document that describes what the sponsor is getting. This is a great idea if you have the time, and if you are worried about *blowback* if something goes wrong. It's like a contract between the designer and sponsor. This can be restrictive on the designer and may

---

[32] See, for example, Perla, 2012; Caffrey 2019; Tekinbas, Katie (25 Dec 2003). *Rules of Play: Game design fundamentals.* Schell, Jesse. (31 Jul 2019) *The Art of Game Design: A book of lenses.* Sabin, Phil (19 Jan 2012). *Simulating War: Studying conflict through simulation games.*

[33] Burns, Sean (ed.) *War Gamer's Handbook.* [sic] Naval War College. Undated. https://usnwc.edu/Research-and-Wargaming/Wargaming/Publications-and-Journals

limit their ability to be creative in their problem solution. It can also remove the designer's point of view from the game.

Another, more flexible, way is to use the "five whys" technique advocated by Stephen Downes-Martin:[34]

- What do you want?
- Why do you want it?
- Why don't you already have it?
- What are you going to do with it if you get it?
- How long are you going to be in this job?

This is a great tool for interrogating the sponsor in order to understand what it is, exactly, they are trying to accomplish. And for defining what kind of impact the game will have. It is not simply what the sponsor wants to do, but what they are not telling you about why they want to do it.

In most situations where people are willing to pay for a game there is also a hidden agenda. Even in something relatively straightforward like a homeland security training game for the Incident Command System (ICS)[35] there are many different agendas that can come into play. At the sponsor level the Department may be trying to get local authorities to realize that their communications systems are incompatible and that they should be applying for grants for that instead of grants for vehicles. At the local level the police and fire departments may not get along, and the mayor and his emergencies services manager would really like to see how that plays out at a major incident.

In almost any situation where people have to make decisions there will be conflicts, agendas, and hidden information. If you as the designer know what those are, either from the participants or by sleuthing (pre-game research), you will be able to design a better game.

Players

We have already talked a bit about players. Most of the time you, as the designer, will not be responsible for picking your players. You may be able to define what you need, or reject certain players, but you won't be the one issuing invitations.

Disease-response games draw a unique set of players, ranging from epidemiologists to medical personnel to emergency responders. Each of these types of players has some unique characteristics it's worth knowing about.

- *Epidemiologists*, led by the M.D./M.Ph.,[36] are the strike force of the public health response process. They will be the ones attempting to identify the index case, tracing out the disease, and building models of how the disease spreads. They are the smartest people in the room and will be an important player in any operational to strategic level game. But, like first responders, they are often too busy to play in games.
- *Medical doctors and nurses.* Medical personnel fall into several different categories. Clinicians and surgeons can and often do play in disease-response games. It's not their primary function but they are generally knowledgeable and can be relied on to help out in a game. Doctors and nurses representing the Uniformed Public Health Service will know a lot more about the inner workings of HHS and CDC, and often represent HHS at the operational layer in operations centers. They are reliable and highly professional participants in games.
- *Administrative medical personnel.* These personnel usually come from the hospital care system and represent the administration of various types of facilities, or from the government where they have the role of administering health systems.

---

[34] The list of questions has been modified and added to in the time since it was first published, by both here and Peter Perla. Stephen Downes-Martin advocates carefully selecting the people you are going to ask the questions, and carefully constructing the content of the questions. My interpretation of this is that you have to listen to the answers and make sure you are digging down to the real objective, not just the easy one. See, for example, Downes-Martin, S. (2014) "Your Boss, Players, and Sponsor: The Three Witches of War Gaming [sic]," *Naval War College Review* 67:1.

[35] https://www.fema.gov/incident-command-system-resources

[36] Medical Doctor, Masters of Public Health

- *Emergency responders* include both police and fire, as well as deployable medical teams such as DMAT and DMORT[37] personnel. These personnel are often difficult to get in games, as they continuously operate and usually have other tasks. They can be difficult to include in games for a variety of reasons. For example, because they are accustomed to active learning a game where they are just sitting around a table can be less than thrilling for them. Movement, action, and active engagement can be important when dealing with these professionals.

Scenario

The scenario is just about the whole game when it comes to disease response. Unless you are dealing with a terrorist scenario, the "opposition" in disease-response games falls into two categories:

- The disease, which is something the designer generally controls, though having a player represent the disease is not as farfetched and idea as it sounds.

- All of the other organizations involved in the game. If you are beginning to get the impression that most disease-response games are really organizational games where different departments work out their issues, you are correct. The old maxim, "We have met the enemy and they are us" applies to these games.

Since you don't really have an opposition in disease-response games it will be up to you as the designer to set the challenges for the players, and the overall pace of the game. How the disease evolves will be up to you. We cover this aspect of scenario development throughout the rest of this book. In disease-response games the scenario carries a lot more weight than in many other games.

How the scenario is constructed, how the disease presents and progresses, and which treatments work will determine how the players engage with the game, how hard the problem is, and whether you get buy-in from the players and others about the accuracy of the game. This requires more than simply running epidemiology models and providing players the outputs. Instead, you will need to understand how the disease presents clinically, how it's transmitted, and, most importantly, what the timing of the disease is. A disease where the infectious period overlaps a 105 degree fever and coughing will have a very different progression in the game from one that allows for asymptomatic transmission. Details matter in disease-response games. Getting the details about the disease correct is both difficult—because the literature does not always have the detail that you need—and elusive because a lot of the information on disease is a moving target as the rapid application of science during the crises generates an increasingly complete picture of its behavior.

Here we are coaching you in building appropriate scenarios around disease gaming, because the scenario is so important in these games.

You can also use opposition players to drive the game in a terrorist scenario. The fundamental question in terrorist games is whether to use live players in the opposition, or to bring terrorist play into control. There are arguments on both sides of this issue. We can argue in favor of live players because:

- They build credibility, particularly if they are expert red-team players. They can explain their actions in great detail and have often accomplished in real-world exercises what they are trying to do in the game. This lends credibility to the red-team's actions.

- A knowledgeable red team will understand how law enforcement works. In bioterrorism games you are dealing with actual law enforcement players on the government side. These individuals have extensive experience in tracking down bad actors and can be very destructive to a scenario (when they round up the bad actors at the very start of the game, for example). Having experienced players going up against law enforcement can allow for *shenanigans*[38] that you would never have realized would work, which, combined with the credibility of an experienced team, can make the game work.

---

[37] DMAT: Disaster Medical Assistance Team; DMORT: Disaster Mortuary Operational Response Team. These teams are part of the National Disaster Medical System (NDMS) which is largely designed to support rapid- and slow-onset disasters.

[38] In our way of using the term "shenanigans" refers to anything that players do that is not part of the core mechanics, scenario, or adjudication process of the game that can have outsized effects and depend on a series of improbable events occurring. Usually, special forces are involved. "We are going to lure the terrorists out the door, where they will become entangled in an electrified net, allowing us to capture them without risking gunfire that might release the agent."

- They will be able to react quickly to the good team's actions and adapt to the situation. This can take a considerable burden off of control, which is also trying to adjudicate and manage the game while at the same time playing the bad actors.

On the other hand:

- Having a bunch of players making decisions for the bad actors can take a game in a whole lot of directions that the objectives, control, and the sponsor never expected. Terrorists are quite flexible people and can decide to do any number of advanced or complex actions. This could take the game to places where the game was not designed to go. For example, instead of disbursing the anthrax quietly within the local community, the terrorists decide to go national and drive all over distributing their anthrax. Now, instead of an isolated local response, which is what you wanted, you now have a major national incident. This can be annoying.

- If you as the designer understand basic law enforcement capabilities and procedures it is possible to develop a more or less "scripted" threat which can then be compared to law enforcement actions. In some cases, the actions of the Red team has occurred well before play starts, and the function of the terrorist signature[39] is to provide clues and story lines for the Blue players.

- You can always pull the bad actors into the control group and make them part of control. The concept of a player (in this case the terrorists), also being an umpire is a useful technique. Such a player/ umpire can be active opposition, but as umpire they know the constraints set by the sponsor, so can keep the game focused on the sponsor's objectives.

This last option is probably the best option for most terrorism-related games. It takes the burden of running the Red team off of control but makes sure the Red team players don't get too far out of control and wreak havoc within the game. Or that they do wreak havoc, whatever the scenario and objectives require!

We will come back to this subject in our section on gaming bioterrorism events.

Mechanics

Game mechanics are how the game regulates the relationship between the players, and the game itself. Mechanics determine what the players do, how they do it, and what comes from their actions. Mechanics in a game like chess involve how to move the pieces on the board, how capture occurs, and how to win. Mechanics for a large-scale seminar game would involve how game time relates to real time (more on that later), how players communicate with each other and control, and how information is distributed in the game.

Adjudication relates player actions to results. In chess this would be rules concerning how pieces get taken off the board. In a seminar game it would involve almost all aspects of the game, from the effect that different player actions to contain disease had on disease spread, to whether a terrorist organization suddenly started using a virus as a weapon. Adjudication can involve mathematical or computer models, but it always involves the judgement of the game controllers. Adjudication is sometimes called out separately from game mechanics, but for our purposes we will consider it part of game mechanics.

Mechanics break along the lines of free and rigid. The freer the mechanics are the more of a role human control has in the game, until the game controller is making all of the decisions. This is extreme and can result in a very disorganized game. Even games that lack any formal rules for adjudication will have to have some rules, for example how long the turns are and what roles the players will play. The advantage in free games is that the controller can react dynamically to the players' actions and allow for greater freedom of action on the players part.

Rigid games set rules for how player actions will be resolved in the game. For example, you could have a simulation that shows how fast a contagion spreads in the population. Controllers would use this simulation to define how the disease behaves in response to player actions. This limits the ability of facilitators to react to

---

[39] The "signature" of a player group represents the data that the group's activities present to the authorities. This means that everything that group or individual did, touched, or visited potentially generates a detectable signature. For the entire time the individual or group was actively involved in shenanigans. This includes things like video records, touch DNA traces, third party witnesses, automobiles, physical locations, movement, theft, and any commercial transactions. Signature management is essential if you want to keep your bad actors in the field for more than a couple of hours.

player actions and requires that either player actions be limited to a fixed set of choices or that the simulation being used accommodate any number of possible actions.

But the advantage of having a controller is to allow for judgement to be combined with the rigid elements of the game. An example might be that the epidemiological model is a simple SRI[40] model showing how many infected individuals are in the population at any given time. The controller will not show that to the players, instead the players will only know the number of reported cases. Of course, the reported cases could be a very different value than the actual number!

Another way to describe mechanics is either "open" or "closed." In an open game, players know about the other sides' capabilities, intentions, and actions. In the case of a disease response game this might mean that the players are working with knowledge of exactly where the outbreaks are and how many cases are involved. Closed games limit player access to information. In this sort of game players may have only limited knowledge of what is going and be required to take action to find out additional information. For example, players may not know the current state of a location until they send a liaison officer to work with the emergency operations center (EOC). As with rigid and free game control, most games combine elements of closed and open to more accurately reflect what players would and would not know.

Games on disease response are perfect venues for a mixture of rigid and free control. They are also good for mixing open and closed systems. You will need adaptable control in order to react to things that the players choose to do that you had not thought of, and, indeed, if the players are not thinking up new ideas in a game of discovery, then the game may not be going well. But at the same time, you need to have realistic, fact-based, information for the players regarding the nature and progress of the disease. As we will see in some of our examples this could be very detailed information. But the players will not know all of the information you develop for the game. They will only know what their "sensors" detect and then only those detections that their reporting system reports. It is entirely possible that data streams get ignored, lost, or not reported because of technical or bureaucratic errors. In the real-world disease response operations seldom have a complete set of information to work with. Neither should your players.

Materials

Materials are the elements of a game that display the game situation to the players. In a typical wargame these include the map and pieces, but they can also include elements of multimedia clips and player communications. In disease-response games there are several issues with display that you have to take into account:

- *Maps* will need to accommodate updating the disease data. This is usually best done digitally, though numbers can be displayed on physical maps using markers or writing. This is because as cases increase there is virtually no way to display case numbers on a physical map in the way we do with "standard" map-based wargames. You can approximate it in order to give the players an understanding of the situation at a glance, but in a full-scale pandemic or major disease outbreak, numeric case totals will be more realistic.

- *Multimedia inputs* to games are also a common way to provide context to strategic games. A simple method is to generate newspaper headlines or twitter feeds using various free websites you can find online. You have a newscaster read copy that describes the scenario while footage of generic outbreaks is playing in the background. This mimics the way many leaders will get their news and emphasizes that the disease response is actually on the news. However, there are many challenges with including video in games, including the expense of hiring the actors (you should use actors), the video production crew, and the fact that the script will need to be prepared well ahead of the event. This can greatly limit your ability to be flexible in your scenario. And if you commit to video updates then, because they will almost always be prepared in advance, it can get awkward if the players do something that is different than you expect and have your video prepared for.

- *Player communications* matter if they are either part of the objectives, or if players would naturally be separated by distance and have challenges communicating. Typical ways in which communications are simulated in games include using telephones, e-mail, text, chat or online message boards. This will require you to provide separate feeds to each isolated cell regarding what is going on in the game, and ensure players stick to the rules regarding proper communications. With the onset of COVID-19 and

---

[40] Susceptible, Recovered, Infected Model – more on epidemiological models later.

the need to isolate games have transitioned to online video conferencing which allows a more nuanced set of communications controls.

Materials are often the biggest challenge in wargames and can become a challenge in disaster response games. You should always budget extra time if you require a map and pieces as these can take a while to put together (thought practice decreases the lead time to produce). You should budget even more time and money for video.

Venue

The venue is often overlooked as an inherent part of professional games. The physical layout of where you hold the game determines:

- Availability of resources like electrical, phone, network, office support, and food services. The easier it is on your players, the easier it will be for them to play the game.

- Relationship between players, and player cells. If you can put them into separate rooms you can have limited communication between groups much more easily than you can if they are all in the same room. Smaller rooms with smaller groups also can speed a game along because the amount of discussion and debate increases non-linearly with the number of people involved.

- The number of distractions for you, the players, and everyone else. This can range from having cheerleading practice happen in your venue (true story) to the ability to access cell phones. The more distractions you have the less time everyone will spend working on the game.

- Whether you waste time and game engagement by going out to lunch or you can have lunch and snacks brought in. Games lose focus when players get disrupted and have to leave the venue to do something. This ranges from getting lunch and coffee to answering their phones. The more you keep the players in place the more you will get done and the more committed they will be to the game.

We won't talk much about venue in this book, but what you need is often just a simple room with enough space for the players and few distractions. What you often get is far from that. This can affect your game design in any number of ways, and you need to take it into account.

Observation

By observation I mean both game observers as well as those taking data on the game for subsequent analysis.

Observers are those people who are watching the game instead of playing it. Observers range from neutral to unhelpful in games. They generally have a reason for observing the game. If the reason has to do with not wanting the game to happen, or wanting a particular outcome, observers can be disruptive. Observers can later claim they were "at the game" so their opinions about what happen should carry more weight. Simply observing a game seldom gives you a full understanding of what happened, and, more importantly, why it happened. For that you need dedicated note takers and observers who then go reconstruct the game and do some analysis.

Analysts observing the game are there to understand what happened, and more importantly why, and then arrive at some conclusion about what that means. Game designers and analysts are on the same team and can benefit a lot from working together. The game designer gets an accurate and objective assessment of the game, which is always important to feed back into the next design. The designer can also help the analyst in collecting data.

One way they can help is that the controller and adjudicator is a critical reference for what happens in the game. No one understands the course of the game as well as the lead controller as they are often making the critical decisions about what happens in the game. Getting to them quickly after the game ends is critical, because much of their knowledge is ephemeral and will disappear after a short time as they move onto their next game.

Designers can also incorporate techniques into the game design to aid in data collection. Examples include things like move forms, where players write down their moves and turn them in. Elaboration or explanation of the moves simply requires another question of the form: "Why did you decide to do this?" The designer can also use any number of elaborate techniques to incorporate data collection, from cards that indicate game interactions to moves recorded digitally, enabling the analysts to play back each move after the game is over. Technology can also be incorporated into games to collect even more data, with proximity sensors or recording being used to examine player interactions in detail. These are only rarely used simply because analysts generally don't have the time to go back and review all of the data. Its far more effective to get consolidated data from analysts observing the game as it is going on.

Inner elements

The inner elements of a game all refer to the human and social elements that impact the game. Since gaming inherits many aspects of play, because it is a form of play, we can refer to play theory to understand how this works. Huizinga[41] talks about a "magic circle" that players enter into as they play. Within the circle they suspend their disbelief and agree to treat the play as "real." They also enter into a social contract that distinguishes play from other kinds of activities.

This social contract says that the players will abide by the rules and concept of the play. They won't flip over the table or punch each other in the face, for example.

Players in professional games often come with an image they want and need to project in public: their dramaturgical sense of self. An official will be reluctant to make a bad decision in public or get criticized for it. They may feel that this undermines their authority. This effects on player participation, and player behavior in professional games.

In any game, gameplay, the game narrative, and the frame for the game all contribute to player engagement, enjoyment, and behaviors.

The primary reason we see novice game designers fail in their professional designs is lack of gameplay.[42] We define gameplay as the combination of interaction between the players and the interaction of the players and game system that surprises, delights, and engages the players. Successful gameplay results in a flow experience in the players.

Flow is a term used by Mihaly Csikczentmihalyi to describe an experience where you become enraptured in a task or situation.[43] You lose sense of time and reality, and focus intently on the task at hand. This could be anything from woodworking to watching a performance, but the common element is the loss of sense and intense focus on the task. This results from a balance between difficulty in the task, which produces anxiety, and your ability to complete it. Too easy a task and you get bored because it's not challenging, too challenging and you become anxious because you don't have the skill to take it on.

In terms of game design, we create flow through the dual actions of how compelling the story is we are giving the players, and through the decisions and tasks that we ask them to do. As the players move through the game you want to keep them between tasks that are too easy for them, and tasks that are too hard. At the beginning of the game players will be unfamiliar with the situation, how to play, and what is required of them. Anxiety will be high.

Thus, giving players more time, and less urgent tasks, moves them into the game. As the game goes along players become more confident in their abilities, and have more knowledge of the game. This leads to boredom, so the pace and tasks in the game increase in intensity and challenge as you go along. Gameplay adds to the flow experience by challenging the players, and the best kind of gameplay challenges the players through the actions of other players.

Note that we include the scenario as part of the game play experience. In professional games a well-crafted narrative will engage the players as much as their interactions.

In this sense the scenario or game narrative also has a role in engaging the players and bringing them into the world of the game. Huizinga would say that the players are being drawn into the magic circle. In professional games the framing of the game also matters for how players behave. Framing is the out-of-game narrative about the game itself. A game to practice a plan may be entered into very differently than a game where players' actions will be evaluated for their performance.[44] The story about the game can control player behavior and engagement with the game.

---

[41] Huizinga, J. (1949) *Homo Ludens: A Study of the Play-Element in Culture.*

[42] See, for example, p. 21 in Crawford, Chris. (1982) *The Art of Computer Game Design.*

[43] Csikczentmihalyi, Mihaly. (2008) *Flow: The Psychology of Optimal Experience.*

[44] Formal evaluation of player actions is rare in professional games unless they are specifically designed for training or evaluation. However, as we discussed, players always bring their dramaturgical baggage and often want to present themselves as successful and competent within the context of the game.

The inner elements of the game are an area that is rich in academic potential for the development of theories and studies of game action. We will not dwell on it here, but the combination of medical, social science, and theoretical investigations provide a rich and complex set of information about how games work.

Types of games

One of the common questions we get when doing classes on gaming is "what are the definitions of the various types of games?" That is a very hard question to answer because not only are there no standardized definitions, but it is also virtually impossible to build clear definitions for different categories of games. Games overlap in their styles, and often borrow elements from other types of games. A large-scale seminar game could borrow elements from matrix games for adjudication or tabletop games for display.

Professional games can be categorized by many different factors. Table 3 shows three: purpose, descriptors, and mechanics. By "descriptor" we refer to common terms that are used to characterize games. Many of these descriptors have no single definition and vary between individuals.

Categories		
Purpose	Descriptors	Mechanics
Learning	Exercise	Map-based
Training	CPX/TEWT[45]	Role-playing
Education	Tabletop	Rigid/Free[46]
Understanding	Seminar	Facilitated
Ideation	Large-scale	Matrix
Exploration	Mega[47]/NSDM	Discussion
Rehearsal	DIME/PMESII	Scenario-driven
Planning	Wargame	BOGSAT[48]
Organizational	Serious game	Scale[49]
Business	Event[50]	Policy
Social	Conference[51]	Kinetic[52]
Entertainment	Emulation[53]	
Commercial		

Table 3: Types of games

[45] CPX = Command Post Exercise which is essentially doing a game using all of the communications systems and commanders but none of the forces. TEWT = Tactical Exercise Without Troops is a British term that means doing a CPX but without the communications systems, just the commanders, but on the battlefield terrain.

[46] Ridged and Free *Kriegsspiel* referring to how the rules are applied in the game, whether they are fixed and written (Rigid) or interpreted by a controller (Free).

[47] Mega games is another British term that roughly corresponds to our NSDMs.

[48] Bunch of Guys/Gals Sitting Around a Table – usually used in a disparaging sense to say that 'this is more of a discussion than a game.' In the UK there is a subset of such games, called committee games. Play in these games' centers around the actions of a single committee.

[49] Strategic – Operational – Tactical (scope or scale); we discuss these games in detail in a later chapter.

[50] By "event" I mean an "event game" one where well-known worthies are brought in to create a media or professional stir by their dramatic playing in a game.

[51] Conference games are games put on at large gatherings of people. They are very difficult to do well.

[52] Kinetic in military parlance means shooting things at people, while "non-kinetic" refers to things like humanitarian response and other types of operations that generally do not involve fires.

[53] Emulation games seek to simulate the internal workings of organizations within the context of a game.

These terms are not unrelated: the purpose of the game can affect design decisions about mechanics and the descriptor. We divide purpose up into three broad categories: learning, understanding, and entertaining. Likewise, we order the player activities or mechanics according to the degree of abstraction in what the players do. Games for understanding often tend toward the more abstract end of the spectrum of mechanics, while training games naturally tend to use concrete, real-world, based mechanics.

The table is far from all-inclusive, but it can be used to mix-and-match to come up with all sorts of game descriptors. You can have a "map-based, tabletop, discussion" or a "role-playing, free, seminar." Just add the word "game" onto the end.

In what follows we describe our definitions of different types of games, along with some applications to disease response. This grouping of games is based on what the players are doing, and what the designer or controller has to do. As we will see later there are other ways of talking about "types" of games to include the purpose, or the target/simulated subject ("interagency games").

National security decision-making game (NSDM)/Emulation Games. This is a large-scale game where players represent the political, military, diplomatic and other elements of power of one or more countries. In the UK these are sometimes labeled "mega" games because they involve so many players. For professional versions of this game the goal is to replicate the internal decision-making process within countries as well as between countries. You are "emulating" the government decision processes, hence "emulation game." These games are usually intense and involve a lot of interaction between players as they move between their "team" and other "teams." They can be international as well as national games, but they always focus on the whole of government and have the players making strategic decisions. NSDM's generally refer to large games with multiple countries, or games focused on the US government. Emulation games tend to focus on internal and external deliberations of non-US powers. A worldwide pandemic response game focused on coordination and collaboration between countries would be an example of an NSDM for disease response. A game looking at internal deliberations within China during a pandemic would be an emulation game.

The strength of this type of game is in the emulation of the decision-making processes. Often you will see Congress played in a game focused on the US, which is rare in other forms of professional games. This is a great strength of these games in that they often allow political considerations to be included in games. Congressional play brings in the media and public opinion. The balance between different government objectives can produce behaviors that are more realistic and indicative of what you might find in the real world.

To take the latest COVID-19 response as an example, the idea that China might delay or withhold information about the virus due to economic reasons might not occur in a game with only medical professionals playing. Put in economic, Communist party, or Chinese national security experts and that course of action could be introduced.[54] Likewise the debate over the trade-offs in opening and keeping the economy closed would be better reflected with representations of political parties and other elements of the US political environment.[55] Emulation games can get at those issues because all elements of government are there to debate the problem.[56]

This "all elements" approach to national power is a key feature of NSDMs.

One of the disadvantages is that these games can, and should, include political play. This makes them very different from most professional games.

Why are politics not included in professional games? Actually, they are often included, only not US domestic politics. Instead, emulation games can focus on the internal deliberations of other countries in an effort to understand the issues that drive their foreign and security policy decisions. But including US (or own country) domestic politics in professional games is fraught with risks.

From a game design standpoint, the risk is that politics will become a dominating element in the game. Players in a domestic game know the political situation and may have strong political leanings themselves. Introducing these into a game can cause dramaturgical trouble as player's "real" lives intersect their "game" lives. This can be disruptive. The second risk is that one political point of view or the other is cast in a bad light in the game.

---

[54] While there is no evidence that this actually happened, it is a plausible course of action for a country that would see its economy hurt while its rivals were less effected due to its own actions. Certainly, China has made economic decisions based on its early recovery. https://issuu.com/horizonadvisory/docs/horizon_advisory_coronavirus_series_-_viral_moment

[55] https://nyti.ms/2ThPd6T

[56] And in some countries, like North Korea, the losers in a debate might get shot. Control will just let them get shot and then bring the player back in another role. Don't want to waste a perfectly good player.

Government service (GS) personnel and uniformed military are expected to remain neutral in their jobs regarding political affiliation and support. If the game casts one side badly, and the players are civil servants, they or their organizations could draw unwanted attention from politicians of one or both parties. Even if no disparagement occurs, or no one cares, there is a significant risk that the game will somehow become politicized in the minds of outside observers (i.e., Congress) and blowback on the organizations or their leaders could occur. This is the reason that Congress is rarely played in professional games even though it has an enormous influence over decisions on budgets, policy, and strategy. And it is why NSDMs are generally limited to training or educational situations.

Seminar games. By seminar games we mean any game where people are playing roles, assigned to teams (no matter how loose they may be) and are free to get up and move around the venue. This is as close to a definition of seminar game as we can get that matches my experiences. Seminar games can be large, with a hundred or more people, or small with less than 20. With fewer than 10 players everyone tends to sit around a table, and they become tabletop games.

A large (30+ people) seminar game will have players divided up into teams representing different sets of interests. In a game on a pandemic these could be national teams with or without emulation of internal politics. You could have a team representing the US, one for China, one for the EU, one for Russia, and one representing everyone else. Players within the team would develop a "all elements of power" or PMESII[57] response to the current situation. Representatives from the groups identified as "diplomats" will interact with other groups to negotiate deals and deliver messages.

The scenario is typically presented to the players as a series of briefings. This is how the players would see information in the real world, so it makes sense to mimic it in the game. You can, of course, also give them written material but if you give it to them before the game, they won't read it, and then they will read it at the start of the game, which will slow the game down right when you need it to get started.

In addition to briefings things like Health Alert Network (HAN) alerts, diagnostic bulletins, and inputs from open sources like PROMED[58] are also given to the players. The goal is to give the players a sense of immersion in the environment they know and understand without overwhelming either the game designer or the players with information.[59]

Moves in seminar games will vary with the subject, but they usually have a cycle of baseline – debate – act – re-baseline. The players are given the baseline situation, then they go off and figure out what they are going to do. Once they have decided that they return and tell someone, either control or the other players, and control then figures out what is happening in the game. In games with an active opposition both sides give control their moves and then control figures out what actually happens. This is returned to the players as an update on the current situation, again usually through briefings or verbal essays by controllers. The players then get to react to the new situation that they and control have co-created.

Seminar games can range from the very detailed tactical games involving individual systems such as vaccine development, to large-scale security games like we have discussed. An ideal application of seminar games is at the operational level where different organizational elements are brought together to discuss how they intend to coordinate response operations.

Tabletop games. As far as I can tell the primary distinguishing feature of a tabletop game is that – it's played on a table. Otherwise, it can closely resemble a seminar game, except during the time where players get to "act" in the game they gather around a table to manipulate or watch something. Often those are playing pieces on a map. Hence tabletop games are often referred to as map-based games.

---

[57] PMESII = Political Military Economic Social Information Infrastructure – a common way for the Department of Defense to talk about stuff it is not really responsible for but affect operations. You can also add physical environment and time if you don't feel you already have enough variables or a long enough acronym.

[58] PROMED is the open-source disease reporting system run by the International Society for Infectious Diseases. https://promedmail.org/

[59] In many actual operations the positions being played in the game would get hundreds if not thousands of messages a day, and gigabytes of intelligence and other data would be produced. The players would also likely have a real-world staff to sort through a lot of it and bring to their attention the important pieces of information. In the seminar game control plays the role of that staff, providing the update briefings from the vast mass of information accumulating at the lower levels.

For disease response there could be several different situations where a map is used. The easiest to envision is a game with a transmissible disease, where the incidence of disease is displayed on the map.[60] The location of teams, treatment sites, and other features would also be displayed. Example 1 used a display of a typical vaccination clinic as part of the game. In this case controllers would use the display to keep track of patients, providers, and other personnel as they moved around in the facility.

Tabletop games are often simply smaller seminar games. There isn't a map, but the players sit around a table (hence, "tabletop"). Control moves around the table and asks the players what they are going to do in response to the current situation. In the best cases of this sort of game the control is very dynamic – they adjust the flow of the game according to player decisions and what is being discussed. They don't just go around the table but choose the next play carefully and use their questions or setup to increase the dynamics and complexity of the game.

The policy/awareness game/conference game. This type of game, like the NSDM, is unique to the strategic level. And there really is no good term that describes it. What it represents is a bunch of very senior decision-makers, often retired, as the players. These players discuss what they would do if confronted with the circumstances of the scenario. In some cases, control then arbitrarily advances the game, and the worthies comment again. In other cases, control plays dynamically and reacts to the player's decisions.

These games generally are designed to be viewed or seen by an audience. The audience could be the media, or it could be an actual audience (hence "conference game"). They also tend to focus on the "big picture" both in terms of the scenario and in terms of player moves. An example of the larger version of this type of game was the game Dark Winter.[61] It was a large-scale policy game focused on the response to a terrorist attack with smallpox. It was held in 2001. The game had former Senator Sam Nunn as President with former White House advisor David Gergen as the National Security Advisor. The director of the CIA was James Woolsey, the former director of the CIA. The players were presented with a video-based scenario and other documents describing the situation. They debated, as a National Security Council would, and came up with a course of action. Then control described the next situation. Media were also players in the game, thus ensuring that media play was injected, and the game would get media exposure.

These sorts of games, even if they are not as large and complex as something like *Dark Winter*, can be quite difficult to put on. Senior leaders, even retired ones, need to be pre-briefed and tended to before and during the game. They can also have their own agendas, or things that they want to do, which can easily derail the game and because of their status control will have a hard time managing things if game flow gets off track.

Board/hobby games. Board games are generally associated with hobby gamers, either wargames or Euro-games.[62] But in fact hobby games encompass a wide range of game styles, from social deduction games to card and dice games.[63] These games, in our opinion, have limited direct application to professional gaming for several reasons:

- They often are designed with rigid rules which can be difficult for inexperienced players to understand.

- The game play can be confusing. Often players must master both the idea behind the system, and the game system, in order to play the game effectively. Again, this can be a challenge for naïve players. The need to "play the system" can also cause the player actions and decisions to diverge from what they would do in the real world.

- Hobby games often abstract out things that professional players will obsess over. In the case of a government response things like permissions and authorities, organizational charts, and communications are critical to professional players but are often deliberately abstracted out of board/hobby games.

---

[60] Though if the disease numbers will be displayed at any resolution some sort of digital map display will be required because, as we mentioned previously, there is just too much information to display on a physical map.

[61] https://www.centerforhealthsecurity.org/our-work/events-archive/2001_dark-winter/about.html

[62] Euro-games originated in Europe but have become very popular in the US. They are generally abstract and not actual simulations, have indirect player interaction through competition vice conflict, and have multiple paths to victory that players must understand and manipulate. They different from wargames in that wargames are attempting to simulate something specific (combat), and their main focus is direct conflict between the players.

[63] Social deduction games involve limited knowledge amongst one or more players who must then work through the game system to deduce what the knowledge is. It is often the secret identify of an "evil" player who is trying to thwart the other players actions while not revealing themselves.

For these reasons we would advocate that, instead of creating a board- or hobby-like game in support of professional objectives, designers should learn from the mechanics and ideas contained within hobby games and selectively apply those concepts to their professional game designs.

For example, the idea of collecting tricks or sets of cards to enable a player to do something in the game can be included in a game on vaccine production. Players have to accumulate regulatory cards in order to progress their treatment. To do so requires additional assets, also represented by cards. Different player groups may have different cards to contribute, allowing for interaction and negotiation between player groups. Here the cards are being used in the game, as opposed to the game being about the cards.

No matter how they are designed, most professional games should be actively moderated – even ones with rigid rules sets that look like hobby games. Players in professional games may be very unfamiliar with board game dynamics, and having someone to walk them through the game, put it in context of their actual jobs, and relieve them from having to understand complex rules sets will significantly decrease frustration and increase player acceptance of the game.

Chapter 5: Terrorist Attack with Anthrax

In this example, we will use a terrorist scenario to build a very simple tabletop game. Tabletop games are very common in the homeland security exercise programs. The goal is to get the local leaders and responders around a table and talk through a scenario. Here, instead of just talking through the scenario, we will add the element of actually having to respond. This will also give the players feedback on their actions and create tension in the players as their actions might actually fail. This game requires a very active facilitator who will force the players to make choices within limited time scales and see (in game terms) the consequences of these choices.

We will also continue to work with Brevard County, Florida as our example locality.

Game Objective

The game will exercise plans and coordination between agencies in a large-scale bioterrorism event. It will include the initial problem of notification and response, federal action, law enforcement action, and immediate consequence management. It will not cover the longer-term federal and state investigations, nor any response actions outside of the county.

The game will include the County Manager, the Mayor of Titusville, and other community leaders from the public safety and medical sectors.

Constraints and Assumptions

This will be a day long game; it will be held in a venue that can accommodate all of the participants around the same table. It is likely that we will get principals for only a fraction of the day with their deputies staying the whole day.

We will need access to both the state and county plans for a mass casualty incident, along with a discussion with the Florida Department of Law Enforcement (FDLE) concerning jurisdictions and procedures they expect to follow.

We will assume that the initial investigation and law enforcement response will fall in on the FBI resident agency office in Melbourne with the FBI Tampa Bay field office taking over within a day or less. The details of this relationship will be something to talk to the FDLE or sheriff's office about, or even the FBI, as it is likely a national level federal task force will be quickly stood up to take jurisdiction of the law enforcement response. [64]

The Players

We will need to include all of the players who might participate in the initial response phases for a small-scale terrorist event. [65] The players would include:

- Brevard County Manager
- Mayor of Titusville
- Brevard County Sheriff's office
- Titusville Police
- Titusville Fire
- Cape Canaveral National Seashore Ranger
- Canaveral Air Force Station security
- Canaveral Air Force Station CBR-D

---

[64] Again, we cannot emphasize enough the importance of these relationships, timings, and organizational actions to the professional players in the game. It is essential to understand and incorporate these organizational details into a game like this. In this case there is a timed process: the Melbourne office will be the first to dispatch agents, followed by the FBI Tampa office identifying a Special Agent In Charge (SAIC). Once it is clear what is happening FBI headquarters in Washington will likely set up a special task force and possibly replace the SAIC with a more experienced agent. This process will matter to law enforcement players.

[65] Even though this will likely affect 10,000 individuals and kill 2-3000 it is a "small scale" event compared to what could happen with anthrax.

- Kennedy Space Center Fire and EMS
- Kennedy Space Center security
- Kennedy Space Center visitors complex
- Brevard County Emergency Management
- Federal Bureau of Investigation Brevard Office
- Florida Division of Emergency Management
- Brevard County Emergency Management
- Wuesthoff Health System
- Melbourne Regional Medical Center
- Brevard County Health
- Florida Department of Health

Now this is a long list of potential players. You may not get them all in the game, but if you did, you'd have a great representation of everyone involved in this scenario. Going big, you could also invite representatives from national level organizations, the news media and local public affairs, or the response assets from DHS, HHS, or the military that might flow in. This would expand the scope of the game and you would need more umpires (with a large support team).

As it is, this number of players is going to be too many to have an effective "round the table" game, unless you have a very capable controller. For our purposes we will assume all of these people have been invited, but likely we will get about 60% of them at the game. Hopefully we will be able to have each player represent their entire operation, like the Kennedy Space center security manager representing all the of KSC's capabilities.

The players will be coming to the game aware that it's a bioterrorism response. It is likely they will have been through several exercises like this in the past. That is why it's important to inject unusual or different elements into the game, such as the visitor's complex getting hit. That way the players will face at least some challenges they had not seen before.

Game Concept

The objective of the game is to test the coordinated response to a terrorist-generated mass casualty event. Players will know they are conducting a bioterrorism game, simply because they will want this information in order to agree to participate.[66] This will require a scenario that produces a lot of casualties, but not so many that it becomes a national or regional consequence management operation. We want the consequence management piece set in the county with the potential for the criminal aspects of the scenario to migrate around the state, testing liaison and coordination with a multi-site state law enforcement response.

To do this we will need a scenario. The agent chosen is anthrax.[67] Anthrax that is properly weaponized can be disseminated in infectious doses over wide areas. It does, however, have treatments available if the treatments are administered quickly enough.[68] Even with treatment, the fatality rate is high enough that it will present a significant challenge to the players in the game.

In order to build the scenario, we will need our terrorists with their motivations, capabilities, and resources. There are two reasons we need to build an expanded, behind-the-scenes, narrative for the terrorists. First, law

---

[66] There is a common trope that players' who have advanced knowledge will somehow have an advantage in the game. Based on a lot of practical experience that is unlikely, most of the behaviors in the game arise from deep seated issues that transcend whether the players know something or not ahead of time, and even when it matters players quickly forget as they get involved in the game.

[67] Anthrax is a zoonotic (comes from animals) disease caused by bacteria. It is not generally transmissible between humans. Humans are most likely to get infected from contact with infected animals, which is why it's also known as "Wool Sorters Disease." Some standard references on anthrax are: Inglesby TV, Henderson DA, Bartlett JG, et al. (1999) Anthrax as a Biological Weapon: Medical and Public Health Management. *JAMA*. 281(18):1735–1745. doi:10.1001/jama.281.18.1735. // Office of the Surgeon General, United States Army. (1997) *Textbook of Military Medicine: Medical Aspects of Chemical and Biological Warfare*. Chapter 22: Anthrax. https://www.cs.amedd.army.mil/borden/bookList.aspx?id=82200b57-a7a4-4160-bb51-4a086dd6ccce&pageTitle=Textbooks%20of%20Military%20Medicine

[68] Even a delay of several hours can result in an increased mortality (Inglesby, 1999). Doxycycline and/or ciprofloxacin are the standard antibiotic prophylaxis for anthrax. Some groups, such as pregnant women, immune-compromised, or children may require different therapies or have different risks. There is an anthrax vaccine but currently that is limited to military and other frontline personnel.

enforcement will be looking for them, and we will need to provide a signature to compare their efforts against. Modern law enforcement can be very thorough when properly motivated, and so we will also need to carefully manage the terrorists' signatures to prevent immediate detection and roll-up (unless that is what we want to happen in the game).

Second, we will also need to build credibility for the scenario. The process of acquisition, growth, weaponization, and dissemination of anthrax is not trivial. It can be quite difficult, require considerable resources, and produce a significant signature to the public. A common problem would be the terrorists infecting themselves with some version of anthrax.[69] This would require them to obtain and be using the appropriate antibiotic. You will need to include how they obtained the anthrax, how they grew it, where they grew it, how they weaponized it without killing themselves, and how they disseminated it without killing the anthrax. Detailed narratives can be built for both of these cases, but, for obvious reasons, we won't go into them here.

Once effective dissemination has occurred you will need to have some idea of where the anthrax goes and what the affected populations are. This is usually done through the use of plume models. Plume models use the characteristics of chemical or biological agents, along with specified weather and terrain conditions, to determine the concentration of agent at a given location along the ground.[70] Getting the plume right is important for credibility in a game, but the ability to model the actual plume in the real world is highly problematic.[71] Therefore whatever you choose to do within the context of your game is probably fine as long as it does not violate the laws of sensibility and physics. Since we want a very small area to be affected (small for an anthrax plume) we can pretty much choose how our downwind hazard area looks. A simple way to construct a downwind hazard area is to simply use someone else's. In this case we will look at an article on anthrax downwind hazard areas to get a general idea of the length and width of our plume.[72]

In the paper I am using a 1kg release of anthrax gives us a plume approximately 20km wide by 30km long.[73] That will, of course, depend on a lot of things, like the nature of the anthrax released, the efficiency of release, the weather conditions, and the location. In this case there was a .44 to .73 probability of infection along the main line of the release, meaning a significant number falling under the center of the plume would be infected. We can also change this by simply increasing the duration of the release or moving the source. Which we will do.[74]

In figure 3 we show a plume that has a concentration gradient which will result in different numbers inhaling a lethal dose. Fifty percent of those within the "50%" zone of the plume will receive a dose of anthrax sufficient to send them to the medical system. For game purposes these are the people who we will track, those with a sub-lethal dose may be affected, but they will eventually recover. This is a very simplistic version of the plume and the population model, but it is sufficient for our purposes in the game.

---

[69] Cutaneous anthrax is the most common form, with other forms being gastro-intestinal and inhalational. Inhalational is the most lethal, and the one that is assumed in a terrorist attack.

[70] An example of a plume model is the Hazard Predication and Assessment Capability (HPAC) and Consequence Assessment Tool (CATS) (Defense Threat Reduction Agency, Office of Public Affairs. (Jan 2008) *DTRA and Consequence Management*. Fact Sheet.). For a description of other models and a description of CATS see Samuels, William B. et al. (2012) "Frameworks and tools for emergency response and crisis management," *WIT Transactions on State of the Art in Science and Engineering*. (54): 293-303.

[71] For a look at dispersion modeling and accuracy see Chang, J.C., S.R. Hanna, Z. Boybeyi, and P. Franzese, (2005) "Use of Salt Lake City URBAN 2000 Field Data to Evaluate the Urban Hazard Prediction Assessment Capability (HPAC) Dispersion Model." *J. Appl. Meteor.*, 44, 485–501, https://doi.org/10.1175/JAM2205.1 https://journals.ametsoc.org/doi/abs/10.1175/JAM2205.1

[72] Buckeridge, David & Owens, Douglas & Switzer, Paul & Frank, John & Musen, Mark. (2007). "Evaluating Detection of an Inhalational Anthrax Outbreak." *Emerging infectious diseases*. 12. 1942-9. 10.3201/eid1212.060331.

[73] Budkeridge (2007).

[74] As long as you get the plume to the nearest order of magnitude, I believe you are free to do what you need to in games. That's about all that the actual plume models are good for anyway. Here I could easily construct a model run to mimic what I did here, but for game purposes this is good enough. Do not get too hung up on plume models, they are very rough approximations of reality, not ground truth.

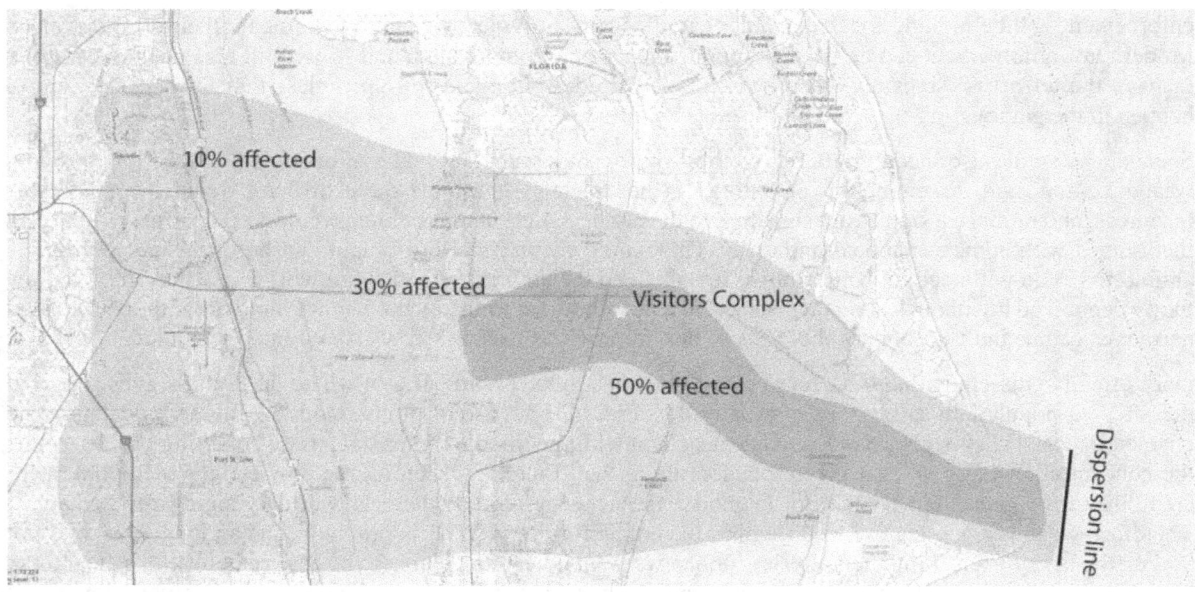

Figure 3 – Plume model.[75]

The plume was generated by the terrorists using a boat to disseminate the agent just offshore of the Cape Canaveral Air Station. Such a boat might be seen as unusual, but they successfully disguised themselves as early morning fishermen and were ignored by base security. They were also standing off by several kilometers from shore. The boat was either rented or stolen (depending on how many leads you want to give the FBI) from a marina in Port Canaveral. If you want to really mess with law enforcement, you'd have them simply return the boat after stealing it, and law enforcement pick up on the boat when the owner came down with cutaneous anthrax. Otherwise, they pull up to any number of isolated take-outs and set it on fire. Either way they are able to lay down a line of about 1kg of aerosolized anthrax. That is enough to generate the 20km by 40km plume we are assuming here. If it isn't, just assume 2kg of anthrax.

In the central area we have 50 percent of those falling under the plume receiving a lethal dose of anthrax. However, most of that area is empty land, so we have modified our plume to have it veer to the north an hit the visitors' complex. This will complicate the response efforts as many of those visitors will go back to the Orlando area after being exposed. The question will become: was there multiple releases or just one? The answer should come from an epidemiological investigation.

Titusville, Florida, has a population of 46,000[76] as of 2020. Ten percent of that population is 4,600. The workforce of the air base and the Kennedy Space Center is approximately 13,000. Thirty percent of that is 3,900. This ignores the number in the high threat area, but realistically there will be a number indoors, some will not be exposed, and some will come from the population of Titusville. This gives a total exposed population of 8500 with an additional 4,000 visitors at the visitors' complex exposed at the 50% level.[77] Cutting the visitor exposures by ½ gives us 1,000 additional exposures or 9,500 total exposures. We will need to parse these exposures out to various entry points into the health system.

Barring any detection capability, the first indication something has happened will occur approximately 2 days later[78] when the most susceptible cases, or those with the largest doses, present to the medical system. The disease presents in two phases. The first phase will be non-specific with fever, cough, chills, and chest pain. This stage will last from hours to days upon which time the patients take a significant turn for the worse. The observed mortality rate without intervention is between 50 and 89%.[79]

---

[75] Map is from Open Street Map project. © OpenStreetMap contributors

[76] United States Census Bureau

[77] The visitors complex sees 1.5 million visitors per year and is open 365 days per year (source: NASA public affairs). We assume that the visitors are in the 50% zone but only about half are there when the plume moves through.

[78] The latency of the disease depends on when the spores germinate and can be from 2 to 43 days after exposure (Inglesby, 1999). This is why antibiotics if given quickly can significantly reduce the fatality rate.

[79] Inglesby (1999). There is a wealth of detail in the literature that we could mine here, including recent experience with the 9/11 terrorist mail attacks, but we will stick with the JAMA article for convenience.

After disposing of the boat, the terrorists will pack up their kit and move to Orlando where they will start preparing for more mischief. But that will only play in the law enforcement aspects of the game.

The game will begin with the first patients presenting at various locations around Brevard County and Orlando. The controller will run the game by focusing on the main players at the particular point in game time, starting with the hospital and medical professionals. They will present them with data and observations coming in from their emergency rooms and clinics. The controller will then ask them what they are going to do given the information they have. Most likely the first reaction will be to do nothing: there is clearly some sort of respiratory illness going around and the front-line medical facilities will likely report a flu-like outbreak to the local health department.

At some point someone will determine the disease is bacterial and there are a large number of patients, too large for a simple outbreak. Now the controller will turn to the public health professionals and ask what they are going to do. They will likely map the outbreak and see that it is very focused on one geographical area and demographic. Diagnostics, most likely PCR-ELISA,[80] will return anthrax at about the same time. At this point law enforcement and disaster response will get involved. And the controller will then turn to them as they go around the table. This process will continue with different agencies and individuals playing off of each other regarding their responses and actions. In many situations one agency, say law enforcement will need the other, such as public health, to assist in their actions. Public health may be able to provide epidemiology to law enforcement that suggests where the release came from, for example. Except that public health needs to know they need to do that.

The game will continue until we run out of time or our objectives have been met. Likely what will happen is that things will eventually be assessed to be under control, and routine operations can begin. This will be routine supportive care to patients, law enforcement investigation of the site(s), and management of public information. In the larger world, outside of the county, there will be many other things going on as the search for the terrorists continues and everyone becomes fearful that they will be next. But that is outside the scope of this game.

Game execution

After seeing who we get as players we will need to sort through what kind of game we are going to execute. If we have the fortune to have a large law enforcement play, then that aspect of the game will need to be included in some detail. If, as is often the case, most of the players are from the medical and emergency management systems then law enforcement play will be treated as a background element in the game.

Also depending on the knowledge of the players and intent of the game, the game may kick off with an hour, or even a day, of review of the federal, state, and county plans for bioterrorism incidents. This is to ensure that the players all at least know where to look for what they are supposed to do. Ideally the game team will also have communicated with the various organizations attending so that the players are those who know something about their organizations plans and capabilities against bioterrorism agents.

After the players are oriented to the problem and to how the game will progress, they will again be divided into their organizational units, with either individual organizations segmented out or clusters of organizations (security, health, emergency management) segmented out. Ideally if we had enough representation, we would like to do both: have individual hospitals and agencies be able to develop their own plans and actions, and then also consult with their wider communities when necessary.

Turn 1

On turn 1 the hospitals and other front-line health care workers will receive information regarding an increase in respiratory cases. Here is where you can get creative, giving multiple kinds of presentations, different data feeds (perhaps several cases with similar presentations are occurring in Orlando or Tampa), and engaging different parts of the health care provider system (perhaps the very first cases are in immune-compromised individuals who receive treatment from the Veteran's Administration hospital. Emergency management and law

---

[80] Polymerase chain reaction (PCR) sometimes combined with Enzyme-linked Immunosorbent assay (PCR-ELISA). These tests have reagents that react with DNA to amplify (increase) it so it can be detected. This allows DNA detection of microorganisms and is a common diagnostic test for these sorts of agents. The "probes" or reagents supplied to make the tests work are specific to the organism being searched for, and different probes are required for different target organisms. Throughout the text we will refer to PCR/ELISA probes as shorthand for having the necessary consensus primer sequences on hand to use against the test sample. We also are using PCR/ELISA as shorthand for any DNA based technique (PCR, ELISA, or PCR/ELISA).

enforcement players will be on the receiving end, and you will need something for them to do while they wait for the news to come in. If there are any sort of detectors around that feed will go into the law enforcement, military, and emergency response chains.[81]

A key decision for game control is whether to give the diagnosis on Turn 1 or Turn 2. I would wait for Turn 2, since this gives the general surveillance system time to react prior to the alert going out.

Players would proceed as normal, with standard notification and operations. The caseload alone should trigger alarms and everyone should start reacting the way they would to a major caseload. This turn would last 1-3 days post-exposure.

Turn 2

At this point several presumptive diagnoses for Anthrax have arrived at local public health or medical centers. This should cause confirmatory samples to be forwarded to the State LRN laboratories and the general law enforcement and public health systems to be activated.

Law enforcement will begin their investigation and want additional information. Since this turn represents only 1-3 days that should be relatively limited. In this time frame they will activate a major case investigation, and begin to assemble a team and command center. Clues as to what is going on can be slow to arrive, ambiguous, or suggestive, depending on how you want to play law enforcement. The key issue is whether there is the possibility of additional attacks. This will matter both at the state level as well as the national level. Since we are playing a county response, the larger issues will be well above everyone involved. You will also need to simulate what is going on at higher echelons, with reports or requests for information. In addition, higher echelons will push additional personnel to assist in any investigations.

At this point most of the law enforcement play will involve coordination both between law enforcement agencies and the medical and public health communities. That is the key element of law enforcement play in these games.

From a public health perspective your key decisions as game control are when to give out the LRN results. An early confirmation will free up resources, potentially before the county has had the chance to examine what they have on hand and what they can do locally. If you wait longer, then the players may just assume it anyway and proceed, but without as much national help as they would otherwise get.

Either way as control you should be prepared to address the common issues, such as prophylaxis, potential vaccinations, preventative measures, and communications. Each echelon, local, state, and federal will be doing things, and saying things, and you may need to simulate the higher echelon response. This gives you some interesting choices if the national level screws up their response, or, especially, their communications and the local players have to fix the problem locally. As always do not forget those other agencies that may have a role, like the Environmental Protection Agency and Coast Guard for decontamination, mental health services, social services, the Veteran's Administration, Social Security and Medicare, and the Indian Health Service.

Turn 3

On this turn the focus will be on solving the problem, both in terms of treating patients as well as prophylaxing the population. Law enforcement should know a bit more about what is happening, allowing it to inform the public health response.

Turn 4

This will likely be the last turn of the game. Here the response should be in full swing and problems associated with crowd control for mass prophylaxis, public messaging, identifying and bringing in the terrorists, and preventative measures should be the key focus areas. Once players have identified the challenges for this part of the game, and described how they would respond, the game ends. After the game ends there will be a "hotwashup" where players get a chance to review the entirety of game play and evaluate the effectiveness of their actions. Players may also identify actions that they, or their organizations, need to do to better prepare for an actual event.

---

[81] Though, again, this is an opportunity for you to be clever. Perhaps animals are infected by the agent, a petting zoo loses some of its lambs, for example. This is a particular indicator for things like botulinum toxin where birds are particularly susceptible and large bird die-offs may be an indicator (or they may not...).

Chapter 6: Disease-response games

Disease-response games inherit all of the attributes of other types of professional games, but they also have some unique aspects. In a disease response game, the primary opponent is the disease and circumstances, not an active player. Even in a game on terrorism the back and forth with the terrorists is the domain of law enforcement, not the medical profession. The terrorists are just another vector, like mosquitos or rats, that move the disease amongst populations. The interactions with law enforcement may be important because they provide information on possible disease outbreaks and the nature of the pathogen, but they are not the focus of the game.

Games on disease also involve specialized knowledge about disease. They involve understanding how the disease exists in the environment, how it infects individuals, the medical effects, and, if its transmissible, how a disease migrates within a population. Prior to the recent pandemic, many of these variables were not very available to game designers. Doctors are worried about diagnosing and treating the disease, while, outside of a major outbreak, epidemiologists are worried about how diseases affect populations. What this means is that the data needed on agents we care about—biological warfare agents or pandemic disease—is not as available as me might wish. Likewise, the data on how disease exists in the environment, and how it transmits including various timelines of infectious to fatality, are sometimes hard to find in the literature. This is largely due to the shortage of readily available data on various diseases of interest.

Take anthrax, for example.[82] The number of human cases of inhalational anthrax reported in the literature is less than 100, and the number where we have clinical details numbers less than 50. And except for the 10-11 9/11 cases, many of these are historical or poorly documented.[83] From this limited data set we end up extrapolating what might happen when 10,000 are exposed.[84] While a deep dive into the literature will produce details on recent uses,[85] as well as conflicting information about its environmental fate,[86] you will not get a clear consensus about such things as fate in the environment, infectious dosing, or movement within buildings.

We simultaneously have a lot of information in the literature about diseases, but we still lack consistent data or parameters for aspects of the disease we care about for game design. Everyone knows their own "right" answer, but an examination of the literature suggests many of these parameters vary widely. Including presentation of the disease.

Also, unlike conventional hobby games, there are not a lot of examples to draw on for inspiration. We have plenty of hobby examples of tank-on-tank combat, or strategic, policy level, mechanics. We don't have a lot of games on disease response. While the obvious answer is "we have *Pandemic*," it is not a terribly satisfactory answer. *Pandemic* was published in 2008 as a family board game. It portrayed several simultaneous virulent disease outbreaks across the world which the players treat the hotspots while finding a cure. It is highly abstracted in terms of both the disease and the response. It is also designed, and designed well, to give the players a sense of the urgency and difficulty of disease eradication. Neither of those traits help us with designing games that are scientifically based and involve complex, organizational and bureaucratic operations.

---

[82] World Health Organization. (2008) Anthrax in humans and animals, 4th Ed.

[83] Inglesby, 1999.

[84] In fact, we do have a case where there were 10,738 human cases: when anthrax was used against black Africans in Rhodesia and South Africa from 1978-1980. Only 182 known deaths occurred. See, for example, Wilson, James M et al. "Reanalysis of the anthrax epidemic in Rhodesia, 1978-1984." *PeerJ* vol. 4 e2686. 10 Nov. 2016, doi:10.7717/peerj.2686 // Martinez, Ian. (2003) Rhodesian Anthrax: The use of bacteriological and chemical agents during the liberation war of 1965-1980," *Ind. Int'l and Comp. L. Rev.* 13:2:447-479.

[85] F A Abramova, L M Grinberg, O V Yampolskaya, D H Walker (Mar 1993) Pathology of inhalational anthrax in 42 cases from the Sverdlovsk outbreak of 1979. *Proceedings of the National Academy of Sciences*, 90 (6) 2291-2294; DOI: 10.1073/pnas.90.6.2291 // Jernigan, J A et al. (2001) "Bioterrorism-related inhalational anthrax: the first 10 cases reported in the United States." *Emerging infectious diseases* vol. 7,6: 933-44. doi:10.3201/eid0706.010604 // Guarner, Jeannette et al. (Aug 2003) "Pathology and Pathogenesis of Bioterrorism-Related Inhalational Anthrax," *The American Journal of Pathology*, Volume 163, Issue 2, 701 - 709

[86] Wilkening, Dean A. (May 2006) "Sverdlovsk revisited: Modeling human inhalation anthrax," *Proceedings of the National Academy of Sciences*, 103 (20) 7589-7594; DOI: 10.1073/pnas.0509551103

Categories of disease-response games

We can think of disease-response games being divided up into games with intentional release (terrorism), infectious disease response, non-infectious disease, medical support to emergency response, and administrative games:

- *Intentional use of bio-agents.* This category encompasses both terrorism and battlefield use of bio-agents. Bioterrorism is defined as intentional use of toxic biological agents that can affect people, animals, or plants. This is a relatively large category and includes everything from spitting in a salad bar[87] to use of smallpox in a nuclear exchange.[88] Biological agents can include "… any organism, or substance derived from an organism, that poses a threat to the health of any living organism."[89] This means that non-living substances, such as the toxin Ricin, are included as biological threats because they are derived from living organisms. In the case of Ricin, plants. As we have discussed previously these scenarios bring a law enforcement component into the game. They also have a unique vector for the disease, the terrorists, one that can be far more unpredictable than a naturally occurring outbreak. This means the coordination and collaboration will be different for this sort of game. And it means that the medical response and political decisions should take into account that the disease could be disseminated multiple times in multiple different areas.[90]

- *Disease response: infectious and non-infectious.* Within this category there are two sub-categories: human and animal disease response. For human disease we tend to think of infectious disease when thinking of games. But we could game chronic, non-infectious, diseases like diabetes as well. We could also game disease causes such as opioids, vaping, or other behaviors. We will discuss such a game later in this book. Gaming the response to animal disease won't be covered in this book, but response to animal disease is significantly different than response to human disease. For example, there is always the chance that an animal disease can become endemic if it affects wild species. Understanding animal disease is important because many diseases we commonly game, like anthrax, are zoonotic diseases. Pandemic diseases are a special category of human disease and involve medical personnel taking the lead in response (at least under rational political models).

- *Emergency response.* Any emergency response operation will have a medical component. A building collapse, for example, may generate numerous trauma casualties. A flood or fire may generate drowning, burn, or smoke inhalation casualties. Disease often accompanies major disasters, particularly when the food or water supply is contaminated. Disaster response can be divided into rapid onset disasters, like storms or earthquakes, slow onset disasters such as floods or droughts, and technical or technological disasters such as release of contaminants such as occurred in Bhopal.[91] While the entire event is an emergency, not a disease, response, the medical component of a disaster response can be examined independently to understand the organizational, operational, and decision-making roles of medical responders.

- *Administrative.* Disease response operations are conducted by organizations. These organizations, whether government, business, or non-profit, have all of the issues and challenges that other organizations do. Business and organizational games bring people in an organization together to examine:

---

[87] Referencing the alleged 1984 outbreak at an Oregon salad bar. Not spitting, but still a salad bar. See, for example, Török TJ et al. (1997) "A Large Community Outbreak of Salmonellosis Caused by Intentional Contamination of Restaurant Salad Bars." *JAMA.* 278(5):389–395. doi:10.1001/jama.1997.03550050051033

[88] It has been stated (mostly by Dr. Ken Alibek a defector from the program) that the Soviet Union saw smallpox and other transmissible agents as strategic weapons to be integrated with nuclear strikes. See, for example, Leitenberg, M. et al. (2012) *The Soviet Biological Weapons Program.* And Jonathan B. Tucker (1999) "Biological weapons in the former Soviet Union: An interview with Dr. Kenneth Alibek," *The Nonproliferation Review,* 6:3, 1-10, DOI: 10.1080/10736709908436760

[89] Joint Chiefs of Staff. (29 Oct 2018) *Operations in Chemical, Biological, Radiological, and Nuclear Environments.* Joint Publication 3-11.

[90] They should take this into account, but often they do not, nor do they have very effective ways to deal with it other than redouble their efforts to catch the offenders.

[91] Kent, Randolph. (1987) *The Anatomy of Disaster Relief: The international network in action.* // World Health Organization. (2009) *Manual for the Public Health Management of Chemical Incidents.*

o   *Relationships.* How do various departments coordinate operations? How do various hospital systems work with public health and for-profit and non-profit laboratories?

o   *Business challenges.* Insurance is a major driver for medical decision-making. Both insurance for the patient and the provider. How will changes to insurance programs create challenges for medical systems?

o   *Strategic planning.* Given our anticipated disease levels within the US in the future, what should medical systems be doing to prepare for the future?

We can distinguish games that have active threats incorporated into play from those with passive threats. In disease-response games, most of the threats will be passive. By active we mean that an outsider is acting with agency against the other (or many others') sides interest.

The presence of an active threat in a game significantly reduces the workload required of the designers and controllers. Now, instead of having to build the entire narrative by themselves, the controller and designer can let the players build their own stories against each other. It's like have a collaborator on the design, a collaborator who starts working when the game begins. If you don't have an active threat you have to create more of the game and may have to create game injects as the game goes along.

The active threat does not always have to be in direct opposition to the other players, but through their actions they may disrupt, thwart, or change the actions of other players. We automatically see the threat in a game to be an enemy, but they can also be a competitor, another unit of the same organization, or a friend who has an agenda different than yours.

Less is more

In all cases there is one overriding lesson that we have learned from running games on disease response: less is more.

By "less is more" we mean that no matter what the threat, a suggestion can be more powerful than a full description. A single case can be much more challenging organizationally than a million cases. A relatively benign disease that still poses a danger can be more dramatic and challenging than Ebola.

Why? Because the hardest organizational and bureaucratic problems are those with no clear solution. If you give the players the 'end of the world', they will either throw up their hands, because it's the 'end of the world', or pull together and know exactly what to do. It won't challenge them to think through the problem, it won't pull on resource decisions, and it won't require careful negotiations. Because it's the 'end of the world'. They won't have the need to think carefully, the problem has already done that for them. Resources will flow, they may not be enough, but you'll get all of them. And everyone will default to cooperation because the stakes are so high.[92] At minimum they won't be able to afford to look bad if they don't cooperate.

If, instead of a massive outbreak, you give them one case of smallpox and start the game there, they have a lot of work to do. Where did it come from? Why was it there? What are the impacts for the various affected populations? Can we contain this? If the answer is no, how do we convince people that it is serious? Should I give up my authorities and resources for this? Or should I wait for the big push where I can look like a hero? What are my agency's equities here? What should I be doing?

All of these are relevant questions when you find just one case. If you find 1000 cases, then you know you have a pandemic and you can dust off the plan and go. But just a few cases. And they are located in Peru. Why do we care?

Less is usually more *and* it has the advantage of your doing less work preparing for the game.

---

[92] While the current COVID-19 political situation more or less contradicts this assertion, our belief is that professional games need to assume an underlying baseline of "rational actor" in order to have sensible progression and outcomes. It is a good policy to assume leadership, and the public, have at least a rational self interest in what they do.

Chapter 7: Bio-terrorism and Biological Warfare Games

Disease response operations can occur within the context of a larger conflict. This could be a terrorism campaign, or a war between nation states. These types of games generally have biological agents included in them as part of a larger process, whether it is law enforcement looking for terrorists or military forces attempting to conduct a campaign. Introducing biological agents into these situations can be extremely disruptive. Introduction of smallpox, for example, into armed conflict will result in an international public health emergency and represent an enormous escalation of the conflict. In this chapter we discuss some aspects of including biological agents in conflict games.

We are looking at this subject in this chapter from and for the perspective of professional games. We will proceed through this rather complex subject by starting with a discussion of biological agents used in warfare and terrorism, then address who might use these agents: terrorists and nation-states. Finally, we finish up with a discussion of engineered agents as these are often something that people desire to incorporate into games. For those requiring further information on this subject, we advise you to seek out the relevant text books.

Biological agents

While almost any infectious disease can be used as a biological agent, the number of agents appropriate for use in warfare is relatively limited. The agents have to be produced a significant number of casualties requiring treatment, easily transmissible or disseminated, have limited treatment options (high fatality rate), and be able to survive in the environment so that they can actually infect people. The fact that we live to such an old age and are not seriously ill all of the time suggests that agents having all these characteristics are not common.

The CDC and USDA maintain lists of select agents and toxins that present a severe threat.[93]

Table 4 summarizes this list.[94]

Summary of biological agents from the CDC select agents and toxins list		
Bacteria	*Virus*	*Toxin*
Anthrax	Hemorrhagic fevers	Botulinum
Q-fever (Coxiella burnetii)	Eastern Equine Encephalitis	Conotoxins (marine snail toxin)
Tularemia	Smallpox (major and minor)	Ricin
Staphylococcal enterotoxins	1918 influenza (reconstructed)	Saxitoxin (shellfish)
Yersinia pestis (Plague)	Rickettsia	T-2 toxin (mold)
Brucella	SARS-CoV	Tetrodotoxin (puffer fish)
Glanders/Melioidosis	Tick-borne encephalitis	
	Kaysanur Forest disease	
	Monkeypox	
	Hendra	
	Nipah	
	Rift Valley Fever	
	Venezuelan Equine Encephalitis	

Table 4 – Summary of biological agents from the CDC select agents and toxins list

It is also possible that agents we list will be modified in some way for the purposes of the game. Modification of bioagents in the real-world by terrorists is neither trivial nor likely, despite what you see in movies and the news. Once again, "less is more" and keeping it simple will result in fewer eye rolls (less skepticism) by the players, and fewer occasions where the biology of the scenario boxes you into a situation you did not anticipate being in. The most common way to modify agents is through the creation of antibiotic resistance in bacterial agents. Resistant agents become trickier to treat, but eventually it is likely that some sort of treatment will be

---

[93] https://www.selectagents.gov/SelectAgentsandToxinsList.html
[94] We have groups agents such as hemorrhagic fevers into a single category for brevity.

identified that deals with the agent.[95] Resistance can occur naturally, as is the case with plague in Madagascar.[96] Unless you intend to create an agent resistant to everything (like Mersa), your clever resistance will merely create extensive discussion in the game about laboratory results and testing for multiple types of exotic antibiotics.

Genetic manipulation of the agent by terrorists allows for a much broader range of characteristics to be created. Gene manipulation is becoming increasingly common with biohackers being able to edit genes without the support of a large laboratory infrastructure.[97] While biohacking may be a possibility, engineering an already infectious disease with a particular set of traits (high infectivity, high lethality) is not easy.[98] It is also relatively implausible, but not impossible, for nation-state to do so.[99] We will discuss engineered agents in detail in the section on nation-state use of biological agents.

It is also worth considering expanding the scope of biological threats to those that do not derive from living organisms but can have significant impacts on the health care system above and beyond the immediate threat to life and health posed by chemical or radiological agents. These agents could include synthetically derived biological agents, self-replicating chemicals,[100] or toxic chemicals that have little immediate threat to health but long-term consequences for health care. These are also useful tools for scenario development.

Synthetic biology can replicate the function of toxins or actual organisms without the need to resort to biological processes.[101] While this does not fit the doctrinal definition of bio agents, the results have the same effects. They can also be extremely flexible for scenario development as their structure and effects are able to be synthesized to meet scenario needs.

Teratogens are any environmental factors that produce a permanent abnormality in structure or function, growth or death of an embryo or fetus.[102] Mutagens are agents that increase the frequency of mutations in genetic material above the background level. Carcinogens are agents that increase the formation of cancer. Some mutagens can be carcinogens and the two categories overlap. All of these agents can be present through accidental or inadvertent release. An example of the inadvertent application of a mutagen was the use of the drug thalidomide in the 1950s to treat nausea in pregnant women. This resulted in a tragic significant increase in birth defects.[103]

These agents have zero applicability as a battlefield weapon because they will not have effects for months or years. However, their presence in the environment in large doses will produce an extreme long-term tax on the medical and economic systems. They become another tool in the scenario toolbox if longer-term medical and hospitalization issues need to be raised in the game. They are also profound psychological agents which will produce significant numbers of concerned individuals whether or not they may have been exposed to them.

Terrorism

Bioterrorism can be seen as just another vector for disseminating disease in game terms. In this light, the terrorists become the "vector," the rats, mosquitos, or fruit bats moving the disease around within the human population. Law enforcement and military operations become vector control, while medical and public health

---

[95] Mayers, D. et al. (2017) *Antimicrobial Drug Resistance 2nd Ed.*

[96] Welch TJ, Fricke WF, McDermott PF, White DG, Rosso M, et al (2007) "Multiple Antimicrobial Resistance in Plague: An Emerging Public Health Risk." *PLoS ONE* 2(3): e309. doi:10.1371/journal.pone.0000309

[97] Baumgaertner, E. (14 May 2018) "As DIY Gene Editing Gains Popularity 'Someone is Going to Get Hurt'" *New York Times.* https://nyti.ms/2IfT5BW

[98] As evidenced by the glowing plants project on Kickstarter. Zhang, S. (20 Apr 2017) "Whatever Happened to the Glowing Plants Kickstarter?" *The Atlantic.* And that project was well staffed and funded.

[99] Most of the discussion about modification has centered around Soviet-era genetic engineering. See, for example, Ainscough, M. (Apr 2002) *Next Generation Bioweapons: The Technology of Genetic Engineering Applied to Biowarfare and Bioterrorism.* USAF Counterproliferation Center/Counterproliferation Paper No. 14.

[100] Wrighton, K. (Jun 2009) "Prying into Prions," *Nature Reviews Molecular Cell Biology*; 10; doi:10.1038/nrm2692

[101] Schmidt, M. and L. Pei. (2011) 'Synthetic Toxicology; Where Engineering Meets Biology and Toxicology," *Toxicological Sciences.* 120(S1):S204-S224. And El Karoui Meriem, Hoyos-Flight Monica, Fletcher Liz. (2019) Future Trends in Synthetic Biology—A Report," Frontiers *in Bioengineering and Biotechnology.* 7:175 https://www.frontiersin.org/article/10.3389/fbioe.2019.00175 DOI=10.3389/fbioe.2019.00175

[102] Gilbert-Barness, Enid. (2010). "Review: Teratogenic Causes of Malformations." *Annals of Clinical and Laboratory Science.* 40:2: 99.

[103] James H. Kim, Anthony R. Scialli, (Jul 2011) Thalidomide: The Tragedy of Birth Defects and the Effective Treatment of Disease, *Toxicological Sciences*, Volume 122, Issue 1, Pages 1–6, https://doi.org/10.1093/toxsci/kfr088

personnel respond to the effects of the disease. The longer the vector can remain free to disperse its agent within the population the more cases, and the more complex, the response becomes.

Terrorist scenarios will need a full back story in order to justify the terrorists' acquisition, production, and dissemination of the agent. We will not go into great detail on each of these subjects, however, there are some things that designers need to consider.

Acquisition is always difficult. It's not as simple as just digging up the graves of survivors of the 1918 flu and hoping for the best.[104] Your terrorists have to find the agent, identify it, and move it back to the lab all without getting caught (or infected and die)

Having it sold to them by a nation state is certainly the easiest, but also the most problematic, route. Nation states are naturally reluctant to put a weapon of mass destruction in the hands of someone who is not under their direct control because the consequences could be unfortunate. And everyone still has to evade detection, often by more than one agency, and get it back to the lab. And they have to avoid infecting themselves throughout the process.

Production is an activity that will leave a detectable signature that can be collected by intelligence or law enforcement. You don't just grow stuff in vats behind the garage and expect weapons grade agent to come out of it.[105] The production facilities will need to be clean and secure at minimum, so that fratricide does not occur. While some agents such as anthrax have prophylaxis, others, such as toxins, may not, or the prophylaxis may not be readily available. The risks of exposure during the entire process are real, and then once someone is exposed you now have the complicated problem of how to dispose of the victim's remains.

The media and other materials required for growth will produce a signature. The more complex the agent, such as viruses, the larger the amount of material support will be required and the greater the possibility someone will notice. There are ways to get around all of this, but they are something you will have to build into your scenario.[106]

Dissemination is the most underrated aspect of biological warfare and needs to be handled with care. Finding an efficient dissemination method that does not scream "I'm disseminating a biological agent" will be something that requires thought and pre-planning. Seeking help from engineers experienced in weapons design, if possible, is the best way to develop a good scenario. Otherwise consulting a bioengineer will be a good backup. In most cases keeping it all simple and remembering to control signatures so that law enforcement players don't shut down your game by arresting the suspects before the agent is disseminated, will be the best course.

Terrorist attacks are different from naturally occurring outbreaks in a number of ways. These include:

- *Location.* In a natural disease outbreak, there is usually an "index case" or the first case becoming infected with the disease. This case may never actually present for medical care and may never be known. For example, the first case with COVID-19 or AIDS.[107] But eventually the location of the origin of the disease can be traced back. In the case of bioterrorism there may be multiple points of origin for the disease. There is the location from where the disease was harvested, then there are the locations where the terrorists disseminated it. There may also be locations for production with possible fratricide amongst the terrorists. There may also have been a location where the disease was tested. These can all be incorporated into the game scenario to create complex and difficult presentation, coordination, and information sharing challenges to the players.

- *Timing.* In a natural disease outbreak the event starts at a particular time. If the disease is not transmissible there is usually a single point of origin for the disease that can be located, and the creation of new cases stopped. Even if that point of origin is a disease vector or water supply. In the case of terrorist use the terrorists may continue to disperse the disease throughout the game period, producing

---

[104] Kolata, G. (2011) *Flu: The Story of the Great Influenza Pandemic of 1918 and the Virus that Caused It.*

[105] Though I am certain someone experienced in the biological weapons program could probably come up with such a scenario.

[106] No, I am not going into detail on acquisition, production or dissemination. If you are not a chemical engineer or biochemist (or both) then talk to one about the physics, biology, and engineering of the problem. If you do not have experience working with law enforcement, then you definitely need to involve people with recent law enforcement experience in your scenario development.

[107] Boni, M. et al. (29 Mar 2020) "Evolutionary origins of the SARS-CoV-2 sarbecovirus lineage responsible for the COVID-19 pandemic," *bioRxiv preprint.* https://doi.org/10.1101/2020.03.30.015008 and Moore, J. (2004) "The puzzling origin of AIDS," *American Scientist.* 92:540-547.

new outbreaks at different, or the same location. Until they are caught there is always the risk that the disease will continue to be disseminated until the terrorists commit fratricide, run out of agent, or get caught. The only way to know that the terrorists have finished is if they get caught or are found as victims of the agent.

- *Target population.* It is possible in a bioterrorism attack scenario to segment the target population. The easiest way is to control the bulk of the release of agent to a particular building or location. The amount of agent, whether it is contained, and the local weather conditions are all under control of the scenario designer and can be used to affect the decisions given to the players. Note that I do not mean genetic targeting of particular populations. That should be avoided as it is problematic for a lot of reasons.[108]

The signature of each of these areas will provide an opportunity for law enforcement to identify the suspected terrorists and begin to roll them up.[109] The ability for the terrorists to move around will give you the ability to have a bigger, or smaller, effect depending on how clean they are with their signature and how long they have to continue dissemination. And the type and nature of the disease will determine how stressed the medical system is.

It is easy to construct a mass dissemination with a very persistent and lethal agent that presents an almost insurmountable problem to the system. But, continuing with my theme that "less is more:" unless you intend to examine that case, I would avoid it. The question to ask as a designer is: what is the minimum you need to do to have the effect you desire? As I have said, that is often more interesting for the players, and the designer, than the maximum scenario. Minimizing all of the variables except one is another way to build tension and interest in the game without overwhelming the players. Remember, in the real world we sometimes confront massive disasters we cannot effectively respond to. But those do not happen very often.

Biological warfare

The use of biological agents by nation-states is proscribed under the Biological Weapons Convention (BWC) and generally frowned on by all decent people.[110] However, as noted by Caves and Carus in their paper, the information environment that nation states operate in has grown murky since the ratification of the BWC, and biological weapons may be harder to attribute than other types of weapons.[111] It is also commonly accepted that some nation states have continued their biological programs even after signing the BWC. The excuse is that they are developing countermeasures rather than offensive weapons.[112]

The trend towards gray zone conflict[113] and ambiguous warfare suggests we need to consider two kinds of uses of bioweapons—use as part of a declared international conflict where one side either ignores (North Korea) or flouts (Russia) the BWC or use in ways that are deniable as part of a larger gray zone operation.

Use of biological weapons in conventional conflict has been relatively rare, and ineffective. German saboteurs in World War I using glanders to infect the US horse population is an example of its less than stellar application in conventional war.[114] The primary reason for this is the physics of the weapon. Bio agents almost invariably take time to act, are fragile in the environment, and are indiscriminate as to whom they affect. This does not make them very good battlefield weapons. These are the reasons almost country banned them.

---

[108] The capability usually associated with this sort of thing is the use of the CRISPR (Clustered Regularly Interspaced Short Palindromic Repeats) gene editing technique. We will discuss CRISPR later, but not in the context of targeting populations. In general, this sort of 'shenanigan' should be avoided in scenario development. While it might (and I do mean might) be possible it fails the plausibility test. And there are usually a lot of other ways of getting to the decisions that need to be made without requiring the terrorists to have 10 PhD's in biochemistry and work for 2 years on the agent.

[109] There are a remarkable number of forensic tools that can be brough to bear in order to identify the origin of an agent and ultimately identify the terrorists. See, for example, Budowle, Bruce et. al. (eds.). (2011) *Microbial Forensics.*

[110] https://www.un.org/disarmament/wmd/bio/

[111] Caves, J. and S. Carus. (2014) *The Future of Weapons of Mass Destruction: Their Nature and Role in 2030.* National Defense University. Occasional Paper 10.

[112] For a list of the usual suspects see: https://www.armscontrol.org/factsheets/cbwprolif. The most commonly states thought to have programs are China, Cuba, Egypt, India, Iran, Israel, Libya, North Korea, Russia, Syria (ricin), and the United States (based on Russian accusations about our defensive program).

[113] Russian operations in the Ukraine are the genesis of the term "gray zone" operation. See, for example, Kapusta, P. (Oct-Dec 2015) "The Gray Zone" *Special Warfare.* pp. 19-25.

[114] Carus, W. Seth. (2015) "The History of Biological Weapons Use: What we Know and What we Don't," *Health Security*, 13:4 DOI: 10.1089/hs.2014.0092

Even something like a toxin will be less than stable in the environment, meaning it is not very effective at denying an area to the enemy. The most rapidly acting toxin's effects will be felt over hours or days, and not evenly by everyone exposed. This leaves the rather irritated enemy plenty of time to strike back at you.

If dispersed into the air, the BW agent has all of the battlefield problems experienced by non-persistent chemical agents: it drifts on the breeze, dilutes as it rises in the air column, can scatter to places you don't want it to, and can drift back onto your own positions. This can limit your ability to target specific positions or formations with the agent, making its coordination with other battlefield maneuver and fires difficult.

In the case of infectious disease, the disease could easily spread to your own forces, unless there is an easy, safe, and effective treatment. In which case you are simply betting on the inefficiency of the enemies' medical services to dispense treatment.

Use of biologicals is more of a terror weapon against civilian populations. They are particularly effective if you ignore the possible cross infection from infectious agents. Infecting a civilian population will result in an inward focus on treatment of the population, potentially distracting from the battlefield. Civilian populations will be older and sicker than military forces and thus generally more vulnerable. It may also affect the country's "will to fight." Of course, this gambit can backfire with their use against civilian populations being seen as a significant escalation as well as a major war crime.

If, in some bizarre turn of events, a game design is all about battlefield use of agents, then you would need to include them in your conventional game. You can identify affected troop formations using downwind hazard models and generate the appropriate number of casualties. Just be sure to watch the timeline of the agent and its medical presentation, including rare or unusual presentations. If you have a population of 1000 receiving an infectious dose then some effects seen at the 1:1000 level may occur.

Casualties will depend on detection and the effectiveness of warning for donning protective gear, as well as the ability of the affected force to provide treatment or vaccination. Detectors for BW should be viewed with skepticism and generally are "detect to treat" not "detect to warn." Also realize that some small percentage of vaccinated or prophylaxed troops will still get the disease.[115] The consequences will depend on the number of casualties, but no matter what happens the medical system will come into play in a substantial way. There may also be fallout for host nation consequence-management support, as civilians may also have been affected. Increasing the overall resistance of the force, including allied and partner forces, will be a major task in the wake of a release.

For games at the strategic level the focus will be on the logistics of the problem, the host nation, and the overall response framework. How will we re-task the force to support whatever medical requirements are imposed by the attack? How do we minimize own force, partner force, and civilian casualties? What is the host nation's response, and how do we manage that? What is the response going to be? Retaliation? Condemnation? Punitive?

All of these strategic questions are brought into play with the introduction of BW into a conventional conflict. If the conflict is with a nuclear power then retaliation and response have added challenges. It will be important to identify before the game whether the game can progress past the nuclear threshold, or if the players are required to solve the problem without resorting to nuclear weapons use. Introduction of a nuclear response, and the potential retaliation by a nuclear power, imposes its own requirements on the game design.

If, on the other hand, BW agents are introduced into a conventional conflict in a surreptitious or deniable way, the game changes dramatically. The exact scenario depends on the type and amount of agent. Small amounts meant to intimidate will focus on de-escalation and attacking the delivery means. Large amounts begin to shift the game over into a consequence management game, although one with an ongoing armed conflict as part of the environment. In either case a lot of pressure will be put on the intelligence search and reconnaissance (ISR) system to identify where the weapon is coming from and how to interrupt its kill chain.

---

[115] For example, the anthrax vaccine BioThrax® requires 5 doses, has an indeterminate period of effectiveness, and protects 9 out of 10 receiving the vaccine (based on animal and analog studies). https://www.cdc.gov/vaccines/vpd/anthrax/public/index.html. For every 1000 vaccinated troops exposed approximately 100 will still have some sort of symptoms (possibly).

The BW in this scenario can easily become a McGuffin for the operational players. [116] In any game where there is a McGuffin it will become a battle between the controller and the players as to when or whether the McGuffin is found. You can control this a little bit by defining exactly how the agent is produced, transported, stored and disseminated, creating the signatures for each of those activities, and giving the ISR system a chance to detect those. In the case of a sensible nation state many of these signatures will be well covered by military deception operations and false information. Sorting through this will be the challenge for the players. The level of detail and the amount of time spent chasing the BW agent will depend on the nature of the game and the sponsor objectives. It could easily dominate in a game focused on regular and special forces support to a partner power encountering gray zone operations, while it could be just another reconnaissance feed into a game where the primary focus is brigade level maneuver in the field.

Engineered weapons

Once nation states become involved the conversation inevitably turns to engineered bio-weapons. Engineered weapons[117] can be required as part of the game objectives. If you want to include engineered agents constructed by nation states in your games a good place to start is by looking at the reported modifications made by the Soviets and extrapolating from there.[118] The combination of artificiality and inability of players to affect the situation can push the discomfort of the players to the point where they no longer engage in the game. In other words, the players will be very irritated.

Gene manipulation can occur naturally or artificially. We have seen the development of naturally occurring antibiotic resistance in *Y. pestis* already. By exposing bacteria to multiple rounds of antibiotics we can create antibiotic resistant bacteria.[119] But it is the deliberate use of genetic engineering techniques that gets the most attention in changing the nature of disease.

Engineering bioweapons can be divided into issues associated with the agent, and issues associated with targeting.

New agents can either be created from existing agents or from scratch. Given the complexity of synthetic biology it would seem that modifying existing agents would be the easier route, but remember you have to acquire one or more existing agents along with their molecular structure before you can start with a modification. Synthetic biology would only require knowing the structure of your target organism and acquiring the building blocks. From a practical perspective it's probably equally complex, time consuming, and signature producing.

This process of building either a modified or synthetic weapon could become a stand-alone game. The players would need to put together the correct laboratory and equipment, along with skilled personnel, source material, and reagents. They would need to do this on a budget, while avoiding getting caught. This would apply whether they were a nation-state or terrorists. You could even extend this process to weaponization and storage. Storage of a weaponized, synthetic, agent would require significant security both physical and biological lest the weapon get out into the wrong hands, or just escape containment.

When considering modified or engineered weapons some interesting characteristics are possible:[120]

- *Binary agents.* The agent is composed of two parts, say a bacteria and plasmid which individually are harmless but when combined the plasmid amplifies an adverse characteristic of the bacteria such as antibiotic resistance. You could, in fact, conceive of a tunable set of bacteria where different sets of plasmids or other reagents would enable the manufacturer to "dial in" various traits such as infectivity,

---

[116] A McGuffin is an object, device, or even that is necessary for the plot but insignificant in itself. The classic example is the Maltese Falcon in the movie of the same name. In this case BW will likely have only a marginal effect on the battlefield but will become the focus for player ISR and operations.

[117] Also known as "black biology" because, why not.

[118] Most of the discussion about modification has centered around Soviet-era genetic engineering. See, for example, Ainscough, M. (Apr 2002) *Next Generation Bioweapons: The Technology of Genetic Engineering Applied to Biowarfare and Bioterrorism.* USAF Counterproliferation Center/Counterproliferation Paper No. 14. and Alibek, K (2000 reprint) *Biohazard.*

[119] Alain L. Fymat. (5 Jun 2017) Antibiotics and Antibiotic Resistance," *International Institute of Medicine and Science. DOI: 10.26717/BJSTR.2017.01.000117*

[120] Block, S. (Jan-Feb 2001) "The Growing Threat of Biological Weapons," *The American Scientist.*

survivability, or lethality immediately prior to dissemination. This could also be done through CRISPR techniques that directly modify the genome.[121]

- *Chimeras.* The mingling of two different species has been discussed for decades in reference to the Soviet biological warfare program.[122] Co-mingling agent DNA might produce a multiplex of symptoms, decrease detectability or treatability, or co-mingle the traits of the two agents. Depending on how this was done it could easily also fall into the category of direct genetic manipulation.

- *Genetic manipulation.* This does not refer to genetic manipulation of the agent but rather the direct manipulation of the genetic code of the target. This would be done through CRISPR techniques where a benign virus is loaded with a gene sequence that is to be inserted into the target cells.[123] This could work as a long-term genetic weapon, causing chronic conditions that extend over a lifetime or even generations, or it could be used as part of a binary weapon, making the target more susceptible to another agent that would be introduced later.

- *Stealth.* Here a modified agent infects individuals, but requires some condition to be met to have an effect. This would allow for a preventative strike to occur well before any conflict emerged, with the trigger agent administered when certain conditions were met. Of course, why go through the danger and complexity of administering two weapons, where each release can result in problematic effects, when you could just save everything up and do it once?

- *Designer.* In this case the agent is modified to produce a certain outcome in the affected host. This could, for example, cause those infected to be disabled for a certain period, suffer psychological effects, or show misleading symptoms without actual damage to organs.

These techniques could easily be combined, with a designer element triggered as part of a binary agent that used genetic manipulation as its trigger.

There are several challenges to consider when designing games for these types of agents:

- *Plausibility.* While these agents are possible, they are often not plausible. We have mentioned this before when emphasizing that in biological games "less is more." Given the huge amount of expertise, investment, and work required to just get a regular biological agent to work effectively, it would be even harder to get these sorts of weapons to the point where they were effective.

- *Player expertise.* In constructing these sorts of weapons players will naturally emphasize the effects they are seeking to achieve, often without understanding the underlying biological and engineering issues associated with achieving it. This requires either the controller to have considerable bio-medical expertise, or an expert to be available in the game where players might construct such agents. Given the investment required if the players seek to construct an impossible agent the question would come up as to what that would do to the timeline of the game. Would the players have wasted time up to the point when they realized it was impossible? Or would they have the expertise in their game roles to realize the difficulties prior to starting to invest time and money in the agent?

- *Information.* Suppose there is a game where you want to examine the construction and use of these agents by nation-states in gray zone operations. The target countries and coalition partners (like the United States) in the game will be very interested in this development. Whether they know about it in advance will depend on the ability of their intelligence collection processes to detect the signature of the construction of such a weapon. Perversely they may know something is happening, but not understand the details. What they do in response, both in terms of increasing resiliency and deterrence, would be an integral part of the game. This means that games involving these sorts of weapons have naturally closed components surrounding the creation and deployment of the weapon. Once deployed control will need to judge how much to leave up to the players to "diagnose" and how much would be done by subordinate commands and the medical community in identifying and tracing out the disease.

---

[121] Block (2001). CRISPR is a gene editing technique that can modify an organism's genetic material. See, for example, Hille, F. et al. (8 Mar 2018) "The Biology of CRISPR-Cas: Backward and Forward," *Cell*, 172.
[122] Leitenberg (2012)
[123] West, R. and G. Gronvall. (Winter 2020) "CRISPR Cautions: Biosecurity Implications of Gene Editing," *Perspectives in Biology and Medicine.* 63:1:73-92 and Gao, J. et al. (Mar 2019) "Viral Vector-Based Delivery of CRISPR/Cas9 and Donor DNA for Homology-Directed Repair in an In Vitro Model for Canine Hemophilia B," *Molecular Therapy*, 14.

Control will, however, need to establish the timeline for identification and trace out, no matter who does it.

- *Sensitivity.* It is entirely possible that this type of agent will venture into areas of sensitive social issues. Weapons could be, theoretically, constructed to target particular groups.[124] This has a whole host of issues associated with it, not the least of which the weapon's construction would be an international war crime. These issues will need to be dealt with in an extraordinarily sensitive way in a professional game. Perhaps the best way is to discourage such actions by players in the first place.

- *Effects.* If the agent is effective then it will arrive as a complete surprise to the targeted players. Even if the players have warning they will often not be able to stop the dissemination. These games become a very complex problem of consequence management for a medical situation that no one has ever seen before. This is a challenging problem to give to the players at the tactical and operational levels. It will also likely change the nature of any force-on-force game to a consequence-management game (assuming the agent has a substantial effect on the target).

The bottom line on engineered agents is that they tend to become the focus of the game when they are used. Since they are unlike anything else seen to date by the medical community, they become a novel consequence-management and patient treatment. They also represent a significant escalation, and indicate that the adversary has the capability, and willingness, to use these sorts of agents as part of the conflict. This can change the overall calculus of the combatants, as well as other potential coalition partners.

In general, "less is more." Engineered agents, while interesting and novel, are rare and implausible. They should be used with care in any scenario.

---

[124] Whether such an agent is possible to construct given the makeup of the human genome is doubtful. You could easily substitute age, gender, or other sensitive characteristics for ethnicity and find similar ethical dilemmas. See, for example, Stein, J. (1998) "Debunking the "ethno-bomb,"" Salon. https://www.salon.com/control/1998/12/02/news_154/; Appel, J. M. (2009) "Is All Fair in Biological Warfare? The Controversy over Genetically Engineered Biological Weapons." *Journal of Medical Ethics*, vol. 35, no. 7 pp. 429–432. *JSTOR*, www.jstor.org/stable/27720364; Brock. S. (May 2001) "The Bugs of War," *Nature*. 411:232-235.

Chapter 8: Ebola

From 2014 to 2016 the US government was involved in supporting the response to an Ebola epidemic in West Africa.[125] The disease even reached the United States. The interagency played a significant role in this response with everyone from the White House to the Department of Defense[126] eventually becoming involved. Because the disease migrated to the United States, the Department of Homeland Security also became involved.[127] There are also a lot of lessons learned from the response, lessons that may need to be reviewed and worked out.[128] Many of these lessons involved improved coordination between agencies.[129]

As we continue with our examples between chapters, we will focus on the operational level response to Ebola. Let's assume that we have a game sponsor interested in the US government interactions that occur during an overseas virus response. This game won't be set in any one geographic location, instead it will focus on the interagency-level interactions that could occur within US government agencies. We will also focus on the policy-making response. To do this we will need to twist the scenario a bit, in order to emphasize the interagency aspects of the problem. And to give the White House substantial policy issues.

Objective

The objective of the game is to better understand the issues involved in interagency policy making during an outbreak of hemorrhagic disease.[130] The lessons from the 2014 Ebola response provide a starting point for interagency coordination.[131] The goal of the exercise is to understand how policy stressors might affect those plans and frameworks.

Underlying the game objective is the sponsor's personal belief that many lessons from 2014 have not been learned.[132] A more stressful or complex response may not go as well as 2014 did, and the staffs and organizations involved need to understand that.

The game will be played by a variety of players, primarily at the GS-14/15/O-6/5 level.[133] These players represent the institutional memory for the organizations they represent and will be responsible for taking game results and encoding them in doctrine and policy. This sort of game is typically a large-scale seminar game where the players represent their own agencies and work in agency teams, and an interagency meta-team, to understand and respond to the problem. Just as they would in real life.

Constraints

Other than a focus on hemorrhagics and the need for a robust scenario which will drive players to complex policy decisions, we have remarkably few constraints. We can assume that we have a flexible venue with multiple break out rooms available. We will expect to entertain between 30-40 players from the interagency, and we have up to 3-4 days for the game. These are not unusual parameters for a large-scale, seminar game.

---

[125] Centers for Disease Control and Prevention. (8 Jul 2016) "CDC's Response to the 2014-2016 Ebola Epidemic – West Africa and the United States," *MMWR Supplement*. 65:3

[126] Dembek, Z. et al. (2017) "Operational Perspective of Lessons Learned from the Ebola Crisis." *Military Medicine*. 182:1/2: e1507

[127] Office of the Inspector General (OIG). (6 Jan 2016) *DHS' Ebola Response Needs Better Coordination, Training, and Execution*. OIG-16-18.

[128] Fielding, J. (chair). (Jun 2016) *Report of the Independent Panel on the U.S. Department of Health and Human Services (HHS) Ebola Response.*

[129] OIG 2016.

[130] The nature of hemorrhagics make specifying the group an important part of the overall objective. But we want to leave enough room so we can flex to the various families of disease as we need to in the scenario.

[131] Bell, B. et al. (8 Jul 2016) "Overview, Control Strategies, and Lessons Learned in the CDC Response to the 2014-2016 Ebola Epidemic," *MMWR*: 65:3:4-11.

[132] I'm making this up. Lessons were probably well learned, and everything will be fine if this happens in the future. No need to worry.

[133] GS = Government Service/O-6/5 Colonel/Captain or Lt. Colonel/Commander. They are shorthand for government ranks. A GS-15 is roughly equivalent to a military O-6/Colonel/Captain.

Players

The players for this game will be the principals in charge of disease response and security for the US government:

- White House NSC advisor
- Department of State; Office of International Health and Biodefense
- HHS Assistant Secretary for Public Health Response
- CDC Director
- HHS Office of Global Affairs
- INDO-PACIFIC Command G-3 Operations
- INDO-PACIFIC Command Force Surgeon
- DHS Office of Strategy, Policy, and Plans
- DHS Office of International Engagement
- DHS Customs and Border Patrol
- Animal Plant Health Inspection Service (APHIS) Department of Agriculture
- Japan
- China
- Philippines
- World Health Organization

Players would represent their agencies as well as their areas of expertise. For Japan, China, and the Philippines we would have subject matter experts playing those countries. The experts would hopefully be experts in health response in those countries, or at least have a detailed understanding. The objective for all the players would be to come to a domestic and international plan to respond to the outbreak, contain it, and build a consistent and effective message about it. The message would need to be consistent across government agencies, with the public, and to the international community.

Game concept

So, what are these complex policy decisions we need to give to the players? We will need the various components of the interagency to have their own equities, or interests, in the situation. Instead of everyone simply going along with what the medical professionals want to do, we will want the various agencies and departments to have agendas that complicate the medical response.

The complications we will focus on are:

- *Security threat.* This is always a good way to get the Department of Defense both involved and having its own point of view. If there is a security threat then DoD may have the mission of dealing with the security threat. The means for dealing with a threat may not be compatible with everything the medical professionals want to do. It can also raise complications with the Department of State if the host nation has sensitivities regarding security operations in their country.[134]

- *Diplomatic and international issues.* In some cases, countries may not want help. This may be contrary to best practices in public health or case management. How we respond in those circumstances, where one country's mis-managed public health response is affecting neighboring countries, is a complex problem and has not been thought about a lot in the security community.[135]

---

[134] "Host nation" is the country who has invited everyone in to help.

[135] Because it rarely happens. More common is the situation where a country limits or manages information about a disease which impedes but does not thwart a response. This was what happened with the 2003 SARS outbreak. See, for example, General Accounting Office (GAO). (Apr 2004) *Emerging Infectious Diseases: Asian SARS Outbreak Challenged International and National Responses.* GAO-04-564. and Hutzler, Charles, et al. (14 Apr 2003) "China's

- *Terrorism.* Introducing terrorism to the scenario automatically changes the situation from a medical response to a bioterrorism response. This creates shifting interagency authorities and requires additional coordination. Merely suggesting that there might be terrorist involvement often has the same effect, without your having to design a more complex scenario.

- *Unusual presentation.* Ebola outbreaks happen all of the time.[136] Sometimes they become large, and go international, as was the case in the 2014-2016 outbreak. An interesting fact we can play off of is the discovery in 1989 of the Reston ebolavirus in monkeys imported to the US from the Philippines.[137] Now in our random exploration of issues and agents we have found something interesting. No one expects Ebola in the Philippines, and Ebola in the Philippines would have all kinds of secondary effects within the Philippines, and in the region.[138]

Placing the disease outbreak in the Philippines, during the present day would have several important implications.

We would need to hold constant or control for the coronavirus outbreak. In most cases you do not want to attempt to have players deal with two divergent issues at the same time. It simply overwhelms the players in the game, unless that is the actual goal of the game. It also greatly increases the amount of work we will need to do as control. Now everyone requires updates on actions and progress of the COVID-19 in addition to the primary disease we are dealing with. Since many of the players will be involved in both responses, it also doubles the workload on the players. Simply using COVID-19 will not stress the players in the same way a new outbreak would, as many of the policy and political implications of COVID-19 are already established.

Since we want to focus on the Ebola response, we will place the outbreak at an unspecified time in the future after COVID-19 has died down to a seasonal virus, similar to, but more lethal than, the flu. That way we will avoid complications with the current COVID-19 response.

We will also need to ensure that the outbreak is significant enough to catch the attention of the international community. We can do this by playing off the discovery of *Reston ebolavirus* (REBOV) in pigs, and that some of the pigs were also infected with two respiratory diseases: porcine reproductive and respiratory syndrome virus (PRRSV) and porcine circovirus type 2 (PCV-2).

The co-infection with other respiratory diseases likely increases the spread of REBOV in pig populations and complicates diagnosis. Its presence in pigs gives us the chance to change it so it is infectious to humans.[139]

Approximately 2 months prior to the start of the game, several pigs in rural Mindanao were infected with REBOV from an unidentified source, likely bat feces from bats living in the barn where the pigs were raised. They passed it on to their litters. After weaning, the pigs from the infected litters were transferred to the industrial hog farming operation, CDR Pig Farms, located approximately 25 miles from downtown Manilla.[140] Upon arriving at CDR the REBOV spread rapidly, and asymptomatically, through the hog population. At some point in its journey through the finishing operation it crossed with a variant of the human coronavirus and became infectious to humans.[141] In doing so it also increased its fragility and decreased its survivability in the environment.[141] Humans also require a significant dose of the virus to become infected. This gives us a low reproduction factor, around R 1, which we can tune according to how severe or mild we want to make the disease. The mortality will remain at Ebola levels of 2-21 days incubation period with 50 (*E. Sudan*)-90% (*E. Zaire*) fatality rates.[142] The virus is much more robust in pigs, with a 2-5 day incubation period and a very low fatality rate (2%).

Slow Response on SARS Raises Concerns on Cooperation," *Wall St. Journal.* https://www.wsj.com/articles/SB1050229161936261840?shareToken=st3fc5c846c4c44925b8a875f880bddabf

[136]See, for example, Centers for Disease Control and Prevention. (14 Apr 2016) *Known Cases and Outbreaks of Ebola Virus Disease, in Reverse Chronological Order.* CDC 41088/DS1

[137] We are going to rely on this paper a lot: Miranda, Mary E. and Noel Lee J. Miranda. (2011) "*Reston ebolavirus* in Humans and Animals in the Philippines: A Review," *JID.* 204:Suppl 3.S757

[138] This is not a unique idea, someone has beaten us to it, but we won't let that stop us: Preston, Richard. (1994) *The Hot Zone.* But we will ignore the bits about dissolving organs.

[139] Marsh, G. et al. (2011) "Ebola Reston Virus Infection of Pigs: Clinical Significance and Transmission Potential," *JID*: 204: Supp 3.

[140] This discussion is based on actual pig farms north of Manila, the names have been changed for obvious reasons.

[141] We don't want "Ebola flu" instead we want something of concern, but not something that will give us the scale and effects of another pandemic. No one wants that. So, we will up the lethality, keep the transmissibility of REBOV, but decrease its survivability on surfaces to give us something that is transmissible, but not highly transmissible.

[142] Borio, Luciana & Inglesby, Thomas & Peters, C.J. & Schmaljohn, Alan & Hughes, James & Jahrling, Peter & Ksiazek, Thomas & Johnson, Karl & Meyerhoff, Andrea & O'Toole, Tara & Ascher, Michael & Bartlett, John & Breman,

The disease spread throughout the CDR heard, and several slaughterhouses where raw pig carcasses were prepared for butchers in Manilla as well as shipment of frozen half carcasses to Japan and China. Approximately 7 days after the initial shipments went to market several butchers in the northern Manilla suburbs began to present with a set of symptoms associated with early-stage Ebola. The variability in the symptoms, and lack of a clear early-on hemorrhagic presentation caused most of the cases to be missed and returned home with standard medications. None of them got better. Most returned in an average of 7 days with progressive onset symptoms including hemorrhaging. At that point Philippine public health picked up a signal that a serious disease outbreak was occurring in the northern Manilla area.

Unfortunately for everyone involved, the ruling government of the Philippines did not want to have a major outbreak disrupt the local economy. Philippine medical professionals and public health professionals were told to downplay the event and seek to contain and correct it amongst themselves. This resulted in the underlying association with pork production being missed, as the local doctors failed to report deaths occurring at local pig farms in rural areas. Pork continued to be processed and exported, even though cross contamination had occurred and most of the hog farms on Mindanao were centers of the disease.

The cross contamination occurred because trucks used to transport the pigs to slaughter were not properly cleaned prior to use in transporting piglets between farms for finishing. Likewise, farm personnel moved between farms carrying the disease on their boots and within themselves.[143]

This continued on for approximately 33 days until butchers in both China and Japan were diagnosed with REBOV due to their working with the meat. At this point the game begins with the WHO indicating that a new variant of REBOV (REBOV-XX) is spreading in the Philippines and Asia.[144]

In response to the outbreak China has offered to send medical personnel and aid to the Philippines, something the government of the Philippines is considering. Terrorists and insurgents from further down in the Philippine archipelago are interested in the disease as well, as are their contacts in the Middle East and India. Several countries, including Russia and North Korea are known to be attempting to gain samples. The Philippine government has requested assistance from the US embassy in disease tracing and diagnostics.

With an R_0 a little above 1 (set it there during the early stages) and 2-3 generations of the epidemic occurring before any possibility of control, we can assume an initial exposure of 30-40 individuals has led to a total case load in the Philippines of between 90 and 120 individuals. Some of those individuals will have exposed people traveling to the US and other countries (primarily in the Middle East) and so we can logically give several infections occurring there. Not all of the 90-120 individuals will be available for trace-out so we can assume that additional cases will occur. While an epidemic model will be useful to give players a prediction of what might happen, what actually will happen will depend on game control, the players' actions, and the game design.

An immediate problem will be cross-contamination from butchered parts of infected pigs. Since E. Zaire and E. Sudan are primarily blood borne illnesses the presence of infectious REBOV in slaughtered hogs will present the possibility of contamination throughout the food supply chain. In turn, because REBOV is also transmissible by aerosol more so than other hemorrhagics, it could create secondary infections far from the initial individuals diagnosed with the disease. This will further limit the effectiveness of isolate and trace, and also create challenges for any epidemic model of the disease.

The presence of the virus in pigs sent to slaughter will also cause concern for the meat processing industry and the US Department of Agriculture. Should the disease be introduced into the US pork supply the aerosols created during slaughter would place everyone in a meatpacking plant at risk. China and Japan should have similar concerns.

These will all be challenges the players will have to understand, develop plans for, and interact on.

Joel & Eitzen, Edward & Hamburg, Margaret & Hauer, Jerry & Henderson, DA & Johnson, Richard & Kwik, Gigi & Tonat, Kevin. (2002). Hemorrhagic Fever Viruses as Biological Weapons: Medical and Public Health Management. *JAMA*. 287. 2391-405. 10.1001/jama.287.18.2391.

[143] Much of this is made up. Would the virus be stable at infectious dose levels in trucks? Possibly for pigs but potentially not for humans.

[144] We use the term REVOV-XX because we have learned not to specify dates in games unless absolutely necessary. Games can be delayed or re-used later. Specific dates or information tied to specific events can cause havoc in the game materials and can be particularly difficult to expunge or update. Better to use relative dates (five days ago) or unspecified dates REBOV-XX in order to avoid problems in the future.

The materials for the game will consist of a detailed (as much as the Philippine Ministry of Health would have) laydown of the disease for the medical players. It would also have general and special intelligence for the national security players regarding other countries and 'bad actors' attempting to obtain samples of the disease. Given the situation, it may be more likely for North Korea to attempt to obtain viral samples in Japan, and Russia to task assets in the US, than to focus on the Philippines. This gives an interagency quality to the problem of dealing with attempts to obtain virus samples.

If the national security aspect is emphasized then samples could be acquired by terrorist groups affiliated with groups in the Middle East, or the Indian subcontinent, requiring military or police action in order to find, fix, and finish those targets. This could also require cooperation from other governments or might go on at the same time as operations from other governments.

It will be important to emphasize the public information and disinformation aspects of the disease. Because REBOV has been in the popular culture with the publication of *The Hot Zone*, it will have a disproportionate effect to other, less feared, diseases. This could complicate the response and shift the emphasis of the players to dealing with it in the US as opposed to the Philippines.

Another complication is the attitude of the Philippine government. From a control perspective you could have the government not seek any outside aid, creating a very complicated international situation, to having them invite everyone in for a free-for-all. In the description above I have chosen a neutral path, inviting the US in to get the Department of State and CDC in play but also considering inviting China in as well. The role of China could also be run as aggressive, with the possibility of direct military intervention, or passively, with them attempting to supply aid and exploit the information environment. It would very much depend on where the sponsor wanted the game to go.

The most interesting scenario would be one where everyone is invited in, with the Philippine government providing continuous challenges to all involved. In this case I might have an active China player, along with an active UN, WHO, and NGO set of players. Everyone would be attempting to manage the event with whatever coordination they could agree to. Meanwhile outbreaks would be occurring in their own and other countries, necessitating balancing forward response with domestic needs.

Execution

Since we are dealing with players who work with disease response and national security decisions, we will only need to introduce the game structure at the beginning of the game. We will also have individuals playing the different countries involved: the Philippines, China, and Japan who are experts in the political and geostrategic policies of those governments. After we introduce the players to the game, and review the scenario,[145] we will begin by dividing the players up into country teams. Each team will sit in a different location with the largest room given over the US. Within the US team we will further divide the team into public health, national security, and military components. If the international countries are represented by single players, rather than teams for each country, we may simply put them into a single 'international' room.

Turn 1

In addition to reviewing the situation and formulating policy recommendations, players should be consulting allies and beginning plans to conduct operations. We will want to avoid any injects or disruptions this turn so that players can begin to establish their initial plans for how to manage the situation. Do not be alarmed if the US players simply decide to do little or nothing. After all, an outbreak in a foreign country is that country's problem, and the World Health Organization.

Of course, this gives control its first decision within the game. Should the US players take a 'laid back' approach to the problem that will give the disease any number of opportunities to exploit holes in either the surveillance or treatment system. Since the players may not fully realize what they are dealing with, or downplay the threat that China may come out as the hero in the situation. If that happens you can give them cases in the US, have China not only begin responding in the Philippines, but other locations as well, or otherwise increase the overall pressure on the US to take decisive action

---

[145] Never assume anyone showing up at a game has actually read the read-ahead package you gave them. Make sure everyone has baseline knowledge of what is going on at the beginning of the game.

Even if the US players respond aggressively, control will need to have potential preprepared response options so that on Turn 2 the US does not simply solve the problem.

Turn 2

Each turn after turn 1 should start with a baselining event, where the "news of the day" is presented and players get a chance to make political speeches to their domestic audience.[146] Once play is fully engaged the game will more or less play itself. The Philippine government will make its own decisions and the other countries will react. This will be both a geo-strategic game as well as a disease response game, so the game play will occur on two levels.

This bifurcation of play gives control a wealth of opportunities to complicate things for the players. Migrating the disease outbreak outside of the Philippines puts different kinds of political pressure on the players. Players now have choices between addressing the Philippines directly, or supporting allies and partners elsewhere in the region. Adversaries can also exploit the situation. What if the Philippine player decides to allow Russian and North Korean medical personnel to visit? What will China and the US do in response? What happens if the Philippine government needs assistance with terrorists and asks for a US Marine Corps amphibious group to come ashore? How will the Marines protect themselves from both the virus and potentially hostile actors? These and other decisions will arise naturally in the game, and control will need to identify them and build responses to them that keep the game both interesting and moving forward toward the game objectives.

Turn 3

So, for example, let's assume that by turn 3 which will be week 3 in our game, the US has agreed to put a Marine Expeditionary Unit (MEU) ashore to assist Philippine troops in cordoning off infected areas. Will the Marines wear Personal Protective Equipment (PPE) during the mission? If they do, then there will be health consequences due to heat effects? If they don't then they risk exposure to the virus. What does the Pacific Command want to do? What about personnel and aircraft moving between the Philippine and the US/Japan? If Japan declares no entry from the Philippines, but the MEU is drawing its logistics from Okinawa, what does that imply for military logistics flights from Okinawa to the Philippines? Japan can be pushed into considering such actions if it, for example, were given additional infected individuals on Turn 2 who had entered from the Philippines.

This does not even consider the effects of the Chinese attempting to provide relief aid at the same time as the US is working with the Philippines to provide security. Suppose there is a conflict. The Russians are identified by USMC ISR within the Chinese medical treatment facility. The US tells the Philippines, who then tells China, and China accuses the US of conducting military espionage on its humanitarian workers. Meanwhile who is going to stop the Russians from leaving in a diplomatic aircraft with their samples? Since there are no Russian players the Russians will be run by control. This, again, gives control a lot of options in terms of how they want to manage the play in real time. If Russian attempts at acquiring the virus are increased, to include operating in Japan or other countries, this could create a diplomatic and security issue for the US. If the Russians simply ignore the new virus, that directs the game in other directions.

This idea of control using elements of the game not controlled by the players to manage the game is part of what is called inductive adjudication or control. It means that control is acting as a player, managing parts of the game so as to direct the focus and attention of the actual players toward issues of importance to the game design and game sponsor. At the same time control also needs to focus on engaging and entertaining the players, so that the players fully engage with the game. Manipulation of "free" variables, or variables in the game not yet fixed by the game or not under control of the players, gives control that chance to manage the game without anyone realizing that they are managing it. This requires game controllers to be able to intuitively identify opportunities, and risks, and assess them in real time. Control then needs to be able to fashion a story or inject in real time to take advantage of the opportunity. Having someone who can create the required injects at short notice is useful in the control team. There is software readily available to create newspaper headlines, twitter feeds, social media reports etc.[147]

---

[146] For some reason in strategic and international games players love to make statements and speeches. Even if those statements and speeches are irrelevant to game play. I prefer to just let them go ahead and have their speeches, as long as they don't go on too long.

[147] See, for example, https://newspaper.jaguarpaw.co.uk/ for newspaper articles, https://www.tweetgen.com/ for tweets, and https://www.prankmenot.com/ for social media posts.

Controllers also need to be able to identify risky decisions, which can be brought to control by players. Risky decisions are those control decisions that, if control decides something is true, will immediately be exploited by the players to 'derail' the game. For example, if, legally, the US cannot do certain medical operations on foreign soil (hypothetically) and the players ask "is this a medical operation?" Control needs to be smart enough to reply "so what do you mean by that question?" instead of "yes". Because if its "yes" then the players smile, put down their pencils, and say that its over because they are prohibited from doing anything.

Chapter 9: Biology and Epidemiology in Games

You do not have to be a biochemist, medical professional, or epidemiologist to put on games related to disease response. However, there are certain things that you should know if you are going to do so. In this section we will discuss the basic medical, epidemiological, and engineering information that can come in handy if you are designing a game. None of this should be considered as medical advice or information. For that we urge you to see a licensed professional. Information on processes, from disaster response plans to public health organizations can be found in the chapter on plans and processes for disaster response.

The thing to understand is that a lot of what is in the literature is ambiguous, not relevant, or ill-formatted for games. This is particularly true for biological warfare agents. Take an example we will use in this book: melioidosis (B. pseudomallei). Melioidosis is a relative of Glanders and is a zoonotic disease of horses. It does occur in humans, most commonly in South East Asia. It can present with a wide range of symptoms and timings. It is not very transmissible between humans, rather it is usually inhaled or taken up from the environment. It is endemic to South East Asia.

A simple question is: what is the fatality rate of inhalational melioidosis? This can become a vexing question with multiple answers. Even though we actually have quite a few cases due to US soldiers being exposed in Vietnam by rotorwash and others by natural disasters like hurricanes and cyclones you can get different values depending on various conditions.[148] Animal models point to high lethality for inhalation, while fatality rates for humans varies with the strain, dose, and complicating factors such as diabetes.[149] But the variation in virulence with respect to strain has only been seen in animal studies and is uncertain in humans. All of this gives a mortality rate of between 10% in Australia and 40% in Thailand. Or 20% in Australia and 50% in Thailand. Depending on the source.[150]

This is not to suggest we don't understand anything about melioidosis; there clearly has been a significant amount of work done on it. Rather what we have is a complex disease, that has a different course depending on the characteristics of the particular strain involved, and the patient. Looking for a single, clear, answer to questions like fatality rates often will not occur in the medical literature. Instead, you will get a range of values, which means that as long as you stay within the range, you can choose your own adventure.

Medical

When considering a disease scenario there are several medical questions you will need to answer. Getting them correct is important because if medical professionals are playing in the game, they will notice them and that will build your game's credibility.   The best way to build medical credibility into games is simply to ask a medical professional to help you. We have been privileged to work with many different medical and public health professionals on games and they have uniformly been extremely interested in the game and more than willing to lend their professional advice toward scenario development. We often can't put on the game without their input on one or more medical topics (particularly effective treatment options).

Medical questions that tend to come up in games include:

- *Clinical presentation.* Or how will the disease present to doctors. This doesn't just matter for a game focusing on tactical response; often the presentation and symptoms will work their way back up to policy-makers as well.

- *Laboratory confirmation.* If the clinical presentation is ambiguous, or it is a reportable disease, then samples will be sent to the laboratory for diagnostic testing. This is done to confirm that the preliminary diagnosis is correct and to create evidence in the case of a criminal event.

- *Disease progression.* Once patients become infected with the disease, how will it evolve over time? This includes things like fatality rates, but also how long patients will remain in different phases of the

---

[148] Currie B. (2015) "Melioidosis: Evolving Concepts in Epidemiology, Pathogenesis, and Treatment," *Semin. Respir. Ccrit. Ccare. Med.* 36:01: 111-125.

[149] Currie (2015)

[150] 10/40 is from Currie (2015) and 20/50 is from Cheng A. and B. Currie. (Apr 2005) "Melioidosis: Epidemiology, Pathophysiology, and Management," *Clinical Microbiology Reviews.* 18:2: 383-416. Note that Currie was involved in both estimates. It is likely the rate was moved downward by additional data.

disease. Some diseases may have different presentations, as in anthrax where it can be cutaneous, inhalational, or gastro-intestinal. Progression also includes issues surrounding susceptibility and how different populations may be affected by the disease.

- *Treatment.* How is the disease treated? For pneumonic plague you would use IV antibiotics (Doxycycline, Ciprofloxacin, or Gentamicin unless its resistant) after symptoms develop. As a designer, you will need to at least understand treatment as treatment will determine how many and what type of medicinals will be needed, as well as things like whether patients will be hospitalized or given treatment on an out-patient basis.

Note we have not mentioned transmission, environmental factors, and public health. We will cover these in the epidemiology and engineering sections.

Clinical presentation

The clinical presentation covers the set of symptoms that doctors will note in the initial diagnosis of the disease. If the agent is a respiratory disease like melioidosis then the symptoms will look pretty much like the symptoms for every other respiratory disease. Based on the symptoms, doctors will make a presumptive diagnosis, meaning that they believe the patient has, for example, melioidosis, but that it has not been confirmed in a laboratory. A confirmed case implies that some sort of laboratory test has confirmed the disease, the most common being a PCR/ELISA assay which fingerprints the disease's DNA.[151]

The best way to understand the presentation of the disease is to use the medical literature to build a timeline for the disease progression. For all the reasons we have mentioned this can be a bit of a challenge, with different sources reflecting different sets of data or patient conditions. Even a simple timeline is not always easy. Melioidosis often presents in two different forms: chronic and acute. The percentage of acute/chronic varies by country and region with 12% in Australia and 8% in Thailand, while most cases in non-endemic areas are subacute or chronic. Whether its acute or chronic matters because presentation of symptoms begins 1-21 days (or "2 days to many years")[152] after exposure for acute while it can take months or years of remission and relapse for the chronic disease. Identification of chronic melioidosis can also be delayed by mis-diagnosis as it resembles many other infectious diseases. And some patients may have an asymptomatic infection that may not have clinical symptoms until years after the initial infection. Table 5 shows the various ways in which melioidosis may present in patients.[153]

Clinical types of melioidosis and the timing of the disease[154]	
Clinical types of melioidosis	Time to clinical symptoms
Acute melioidosis	Less than 2 weeks
Subacute melioidosis	Between 2 weeks and 2 months
Chronic melioidosis	Symptoms go on longer than 2 months
Latent melioidosis	Disease becomes active at an indefinite future time
Recurrent melioidosis	Re-infection or relapse after an initial recovery

Table 5 – Clinical types of melioidosis and the timing of the disease

Of those that present with positive blood cultures (50-60% of cases) the majority have septicemia. These individuals have a short history (median 6 days: range 1 day – 2 months) of high fever and rigors. Acute

---

[151] PCR/ELISA = Polymerase chain reaction-enzyme-linked immunosorbent assay. These are separate techniques: the PCR test amplifies certain sequences of DNA (primers) while ELISA looks for antigens or antibodies (probes). PCR analyses is very fast, while ELISA is sensitive to low concentrations. They can be used together, which is frequently the case, or separately. Used together the PCR amplified the target DNA while ELISA binds to it. There are a wide range of PCR/ELISA systems available, but all require the correct set of primers and probes in order to be able to detect the disease.
[152] Antosia, R. and J. Cahill. (2006) Handbook of Bioterrorism and Disaster Medicine.
[153] Ketheesan, N. (2012) *Melioidosis: A Century of Observation and Research.*
[154] Ketheesan (2012).

respiratory syndrome may also be a feature. Death for these individuals is common within 48 hours of admission.[155] You will note that these values for the timeline of the progression are slightly different than those shown in table 5. This can either be helpful, or confusing, in developing a scenario.

So melioidosis presents anywhere from 1-21 days after exposure in its acute form, likely depending on the dose and the vulnerability of the individual. In many cases the disease will take a lot more time, waiting for years before presenting with symptoms. From the perspective of a scenario design this means that we will need to break out our exposed population into subgroups. Those individuals with complicating factors, such as diabetes or immune-compromise, may present earlier and with the acute disease. Another fraction of the exposed population will present with either subacute or chronic. Something that the initial cases may suggest to the medical professionals – they will not only have to deal with the acute cases, but they should also start looking for and prophylaxing the subacute, chronic, and latent cases if they can identify them. This means that whatever initial exposure occurs only a fraction – likely between 10-20 percent—will develop the acute form, so the initial case load may be less daunting than it would have been otherwise. On the other hand, medical professionals will quickly begin to realize that the acute cases may only be the tip of the iceberg, and they had better develop plans and processes for the less acute cases.

This shows one of the reasons we chose melioidosis as the example disease for much of this book. It is complex, confounding, and quite difficult to diagnose. It creates a little bit of interest or sense of the unexpected in scenarios because it is not a "normal" warfare agent. It also allows for manipulation of the numbers depending on how we want to present the disease in the game. If we want to give the terrorists a fighting chance, I can delay symptom onset several days without much trouble, at least for a large part of the exposed population. If we want to have maximum initial effect, we can have a large number present immediately with acute symptoms. The data gives us some flexibility.

Laboratory analysis

Laboratories and laboratory confirmation can become a major challenge in disease-response games. The challenge of both effective testing and laboratory capacity has become apparent in the attempt to increase testing and diagnosis during the COVID-19 epidemic. Within the US there is a structure or hierarchy of laboratories for diagnostics. At the base level are the local diagnostic labs affiliated with the hospitals and doctors in the region. These labs will receive samples and conduct the first-line diagnostics. Beyond the traditional medical laboratories there are the state, local, and national public-health laboratories. These labs run all of the time and can (or in some cases must) be referred samples for analysis. This could be due to the presence of an unusual disease, or a public-health reporting requirement.

Many of the public-health laboratories, along with a variety of other labs, are part of the Laboratory Response Network run by the Centers for Disease Control.[156] This system was established in response to the possibility of a biological or chemical terrorist threat. The goal was to increase overall laboratory capacity to respond to emergencies. The system provides funds and training to the laboratories in the network, allowing them to handle more advanced diseases than they would be able to otherwise. Since its founding the system has expanded to include not only local, state, and federal public-health laboratories but also military laboratories, FDA and UDSA food and veterinary labs, environmental labs as well as international partner laboratories.

The biological laboratory system (LRN-B) works on a hierarchy of laboratories.[157] At the base are the sentinel labs, the local medical system and hospital laboratories along with local public-health laboratories. These labs determine whether a sample should be referred up the chain to the reference laboratory. Reference laboratories take the referred specimen and conduct confirmatory tests on the sample. Reference laboratories are usually located at the state level and also provide training and awareness to the sentinel laboratories. If the sample warrants further action, they can refer it to the next layer, the national laboratories at the CDC, US Army Medical Research Institute for Infectious Disease (USAMRIID) or the Naval Medical Research Center (NMRC). They are designed to conduct complex or specialized tests and can handle highly infectious or dangerous agents.[158] In

---

[155] Dance, D. (2005) "Melioidosis and Glanders as Possible Biological Weapons" in Fong and Alibek: *Bioterrorism and Infectious Agents.*

[156] https://emergency.cdc.gov/lrn/

[157] Craft, David W et al. (2014) "Bioterrorism: a laboratory who does it?." *Journal of clinical microbiology* vol. 52,7: 2290-8. doi:10.1128/JCM.00359-14

[158] US AMRIID and CDC are biosafety level 4 labs, designed for highly lethal or transmissible agent without a treatment. There is also an expanding network of BSL-4 laboratories designed to increase the overall capacity of the system. https://www.cdc.gov/cpr/infographics/biosafety.htm, including the National Biodefense Analysis and

addition to medical testing, these tests also can have legal, or international, implications by verifying that an agent has been used, the type of agent, and developing forensic evidence such as likely origin or manipulation of the agent.[159]

In the case of multiple patients presenting with melioidosis in Florida, you will start with the physician's developing a presumptive diagnosis, which will probably have melioidosis in the differential. Melioidosis would be highly unusual, even in Florida, so other diseases might be considered as well. Hospital or local laboratories would be called on to support the diagnosis, which might take a day or so. In addition, because multiple individuals presented with the disease, samples would probably be sent to the Florida Bureau of Public Health LRN laboratories. BPH LRN labs are located in Jacksonville, Miami, and Tampa.[160] These laboratories would conduct PCR/ELISA testing on the sample and give preliminary confirmation of the disease. The sample would also be split, and part of it sent to the CDC where final confirmation and analysis would occur.

When considering movement of samples between laboratories the question of chain of custody also comes up frequently. For samples that may be evidence of a crime, note both terrorism and acts of war count as crimes, then the senders will need to maintain positive control over the samples and ensure a legal chain of custody has been maintained. This can include direct escort by law enforcement, or special shipping considerations.[161]

From a laboratory perspective you need to consider:

- The differential for the disease and how that affects referral to laboratories. A differential of smallpox will generate a vastly different laboratory response than a differential for melioidosis as the symptoms and implications are very different.

- The time it will take for samples to be collected, packaged, transported, analyzed and the results returned to the players. Depending on the disease, and the level of confirmation, this can take days not hours in game time.

- The notification and consultation process that will occur when there is an important result. If there is suspicion of either a highly transmissible, lethal, disease (pandemic) or terrorism there will be a notification chain at the national level and a desire to build a response plan immediately prior to announcing the outbreak. There may also be an international set of notifications and consultations that need to occur.[162] This will require coordination with state and local medical and response personnel.

- The requirements for sample movement. Some samples require chain of cold, a constant cold temperature. Others may require special packaging or buffers to be included. Specific carriers may be the only ones allowed to transport the samples. All of these things can slow things down and delay sample analysis.

Epidemiological

We can divide epidemiology into several related but distinct concepts:

- Epidemiological models that show the progress of a disease through a population.

- Disease parameters such as latency, infectivity, transmissibility, duration, and fatality rates all determine the overall progress of the disease through the population. But they also build the story of how the disease moves within smaller subsets of the population.

Countermeasures Center for DHS (https://www.dhs.gov/science-and-technology/national-biodefense-analysis-and-countermeasures-center) and the National Institute for Allergy and Infectious Disease's Integrated Research Facility (https://www.niaid.nih.gov/about/integrated-research-facility-overview). These increase the overall capacity, but the

[159] https://emergency.cdc.gov/lrn/biological.asp

[160] http://www.floridahealth.gov/programs-and-services/public-health-laboratories/laboratory-services/clinical-laboratories.html

[161] You would probably be surprised at what you can ship by FEDEX.

[162] For example, WHO regulations require notification within 24 hours when an outbreak of plague or yellow fever occurs. World Health Organization. (1995) *International Health Regulations (1969). 3rd Ed.*

- The use of data and statistics to build response to disease. The classic example of this is the use of data to identify the source of cholera in 19th century England.[163]

We will begin by describing epidemiological models because so many of the other parameters relate back to the models. We won't discuss statistical analysis of disease as these techniques are mostly used on chronic diseases and can be data- and analysis-intensive which may not work well in games.

Epidemiological Models

Although epidemiological models are often the focus of disease games, identifying, choosing, and managing epidemiological parameters in designing the scenarios is where you will begin to incorporate realistic disease progression into your game.

Epidemiological models divide the population up into those who are susceptible (S), infected (I) and removed or immune to the infection (R). The total vulnerable population is N = S + I + R. Members of the population transition between these groups over time, depending on the Basic Reproduction Number (R_0) or the number of individuals infected for each infected individual, as well as the time it takes to recover. "Removed" means you can't get the disease anymore, which includes fatalities as well as an assumption about immunity.[164]

While this is a discrete mathematical problem, if N is large enough you can assume it actually is a continuous variable and build a set of differential equations that describe the epidemic progression:[165]

$$\frac{dS}{dt} = -\beta SI$$

$$\frac{dI}{dt} = \beta SI - \gamma I$$

Where β is the transmission rate (per capita) and γ is the recovery rate which is 1/(mean infectious period). Note that γ includes both those who recover with immunity, as well as fatalities. If the whole population starts as susceptible, then the first infectious patient can infect βN patients in the first mean infectious period or $1/\gamma$.

The first equation says that the rate of change of the number of susceptible people changes proportionally to the product of the number of susceptible and infected. This assumes that the population is uniformly mixed, and everyone gets a chance to interact with everyone else. The second equation says that the rate that the number of infected people grow is equal to the difference between those who get infected, and those who drop out of being infected after the disease runs its course or they die. You could also write an equation for the rate of change in the number of recovered: $\frac{dR}{dt} = \gamma I$.

If everyone is susceptible so that the entire population (N) is initially susceptible then the number infected in period $1/\gamma$ will be βN which allows us to define the Basic Reproduction Number as $\frac{\beta N}{\gamma} = R_0$ or how many individuals will be infected for each case within the time interval that individual is infectious.[166]

If R_0 is less than 1 then the epidemic declines in numbers because $\gamma > \beta$ in the second equation above. If R_0 is equal to one then the disease will neither decline nor spread, while an R_0 greater than 1 means epidemic spread will occur. If R_0 is much greater than 1 the disease will quickly spread through the population until the population becomes saturated with immune individuals and "herd immunity" is developed. Herd immunity can be created either through exposure, or vaccination. One way to think about R_0 less than or equal to 1 is that you start with herd immunity and the disease numbers decline over time.

Herd immunity is expressed as:[167]

$$p > 1 - 1/R_0$$

---

[163] In 1854 John Snow used data on the water supply and correlated it with cholera deaths to show where the disease was coming from. He is considered as one of the founders of modern epidemiology. Celentano, D. and M. Szklo. (2019) *Gordis Epidemiology 6th Ed.*

[164] Brauer, F. et al. (eds.) (2008) *Mathematical Epidemiology.*

[165] Brauer (2008)

[166] Brauer (2008)

[167] Brauer (2008)

For an R_0 of 2 this means that 50% of the population will need to be immune to the disease through either having the disease or vaccination. This is one reason diseases with a high R_0 are so dangerous, controlling them in the population will require large numbers to either be exposed or vaccinated and drop out of the susceptible pool. R_0 can be a tricky variable and can vary by geography and sub-population because it not only reflects the diseases' infectivity but also transmission paths and number of close contacts, both of which may vary widely.

This SIR model is the basic model for epidemic spread of disease.

Unfortunately, the model is a coupled, non-linear differential equation which evinces no easy general solution (though there are analytical solutions for some cases).[168] The model can be solved by numerical techniques, and a variety of tools exist on the Internet to allow for numerical solutions.[169] While this model is accessible, it's not terribly realistic.

You can also make the model more complex by adding terms. Populations don't stay constant: infants are born and people die of causes other than the disease. So, you can add a birth rate and death rate to the SIR model. This modifies R_0 to now be $\beta N / (\mu + \gamma)$ where μ is the death rate and the population remains constant (birth rate $= \mu N$). You can also have populations that become susceptible again (e.g., common cold), the SIS model, or you can differentiate between recovered and deceased (SIRD), or maternity generated immunity (MSIR), and account for exposure (SEIR). Many different factors can influence outbreaks, from seasonality to local conditions, and the most accurate models will take them all into account.[170]

From a programming perspective a discrete set of equations is perhaps more easily solved by simple spreadsheet techniques than a coupled ordinary differential equation. In many cases you will also have two or more populations with different infection rates and susceptibility to the disease. These we will represent by superscripts, with S_t^1 being the number of susceptible individuals in population 1 at time t. In general, this becomes S_t^i where S is the number of susceptible in population i. We can also add fatality and recovery rates, along with the fraction of the infected population that develops symptoms and presents as infected. The formulas then become:

$$S_t = \sum_{i=1}^{N} S_t^i : \; E_t = \sum_{i=1}^{N} E_t^i : \; I_t = \sum_{i=1}^{N} I_t^i : \; \sum_{i=1}^{N} \mu_i = 1$$

$$S_t^i = S_t \mu_i$$

$$S_{t+1}^i = S_t^i (1 - \beta^i I_t)$$

$$E_{t+1}^i = \beta^i S_t^i I_t$$

$$\gamma^i = \gamma_D^i + \gamma_R^i$$

$$I_{t+1}^i = I_t^i (1 - \gamma^i) + \delta^i E_t^i$$

$$R_{t+1}^i = R_t^i + \gamma_R^i I_t^i$$

$$D_{t+1}^i = D_t^i + \gamma_D^i I_t^i$$

Where β^i is the exposure rate for population i (we are assuming that everyone "exposed" becomes immune and drops out of the susceptible population but only a fraction δ go on to develop symptoms), δ^i is the fraction of the exposed population that develops symptoms, γ^i is the total removal rate from the infected population, γ_D^i is the fatality rate, γ_R^i is the recovery rate, R_t^i is the number of recovered individuals in population i at time t, D_t^i is the number of fatalities in population i at time t, and μ_i fraction of the population in group i. Note that the equations for the susceptible and exposed have terms for those who are in population i and are exposed to those infected in all other populations. We assume that the basic SRI model applies and that there is uniform mixing

[168] Shabbir, G., Khan, H. & Sadiq, M. A. (2010) A note on Exact solution of SIR and SIS epidemic models arXiv10102.5035v1 [math.CA]

[169] http://math.colgate.edu/~wweckesser/solver/DiseaseSIR.shtml and for a numerical algorithm see Brauer (2008) p. 8.

[170] Martcheva, M. (2010) *An Introduction to Mathematical Epidemiology.*

amongst the populations and no population has a different probability of transmission (though populations may have different probabilities of infection).

You could also add in a testing rate, with false positives and negatives, if you wanted to refine your "infected" scores. The challenge will be representing the different fractions of the population that show various susceptibilities and fatality rates as those are not well known. It is likely that the divisions will be based on demographic traits, or location, which are much easier to find and use.

Beyond the differential-equation models there are a number of other techniques that you can use to represent the course of an epidemic. All of them at their core simply solve the differential equations, but they do so using fancy computational techniques. Network based models attempt to get around the assumption in the differential equations (even those with a variety of sub-populations) that the population is well mixed. In these models, individuals in the population can be represented as on a lattice network, or a network that represents the distribution of personal connections within the population.[171] Beyond network models are agent-based models that attempt to represent the dynamics within the population. [172]

How do you use these models in games? First note that, if you are coming to this design problem from the wargaming community, these models are not like traditional combat results tables. The progression of the disease will be dynamic and three are many variables involved that we do not fully understand or have good data on. Often the epidemic is well outside the ability to contain or respond to it, particularly with a fast-moving disease in a small population. Player actions may not have a lot of influence on disease progression, and certainly not in the case of tactical actions.[173]

And player actions will present a dynamic challenge to solving the equations. Actions can affect the terms of the equation ($\beta, \gamma, etc.$) or the structure of the equations themselves (by adding or subtracting disease processes). If the parameters change, you will have to decide how much to change them given what the players have decided to do. If the structure of the equations changes in a way you did not expect—introducing issues surrounding birth and unrelated mortality, for example—then you may need an entirely new model, something that is difficult to create during a game.

Let's take the case where widespread hand washing changes the transmissibility of the disease. This will have a direct impact on the number of individuals infected by each infected individual (R_0) through the transmission rate (β). A meta-analysis of studies showed that hand washing reduced the incidence of respiratory disease by 21%.[174] While this gives us an idea of what the effect of hand washing may be, it does not give an indication of the fraction of people who will actually wash their hands after a particular exposure. There are studies that show approximately 33%[175] of all hand washers don't use soap, and 10.3% don't wash their hands at all. This varies by a lot of factors, especially between men (50% wash with soap) and women (78% wash with soap). But this is what is already happening. It is likely factored into any R_0 that we may use.

Instead, what we are interested in is the change that might occur during an epidemic where hand washing was emphasized. That will be much harder to characterize without a new study or survey, both of which are difficult to do in the middle of a game. Instead, you will have to make a "best guess" estimate depending on your view of how pliable the population's behavior is. A stubborn, distrustful, population may only change 5-10% in hand washing based on a public information campaign. A compliant population may increase by 20-30%. But since hand washing is dependent on a lot of variables, especially habits, those habits may be hard to change, which is why in the estimates I made above I only increased it by 5-30% after intervention. Note I chose these values before researching the next paragraph.

---

[171] Canzani, Elisa, and Ulrike Lechner. (2015) "Insights from Modeling Epidemics of Infectious Diseases-A Literature Review." *ISCRAM*.

[172] Rahmandad, Hazhir, and John Sterman. (2004) "Heterogeneity and network structure in the dynamics of contagion: Comparing agent-based and differential equation models." *Proceedings of the 22nd International Conference of the System Dynamics Society*. Oxford, UK: System Dynamics Society.

[173] Though with COVID-19 we have seen an unprecedented international response to lock down entire populations, which is something that would need to be reflected in the epidemic models.

[174] Aiello, Allison E et al. (2008) "Effect of hand hygiene on infectious disease risk in the community setting: a meta-analysis." *American journal of public health* vol. 98,8: 1372-81. doi:10.2105/AJPH.2007.124610 it is important to note that the effects of different hand washing interventions varied depending on whether education was combined with hand washing and the type of disinfectant used.

[175] Borchgrevink, C. et al. (Apr 2013) "Hand Washing Practices in a College Town Environment," *Journal of Environmental Health*, 75:8: 18-24.

In one study of messages attempting to increase hand washing showed a 9.4-9.8% increase in hand washing after the population received the message.[176] So if 10% of the population started properly washing their hands (instead of what they are currently doing), then there would be a 2% decrease in respiratory disease (because hand washing decreases incidents of disease by 21% as described above). This is not a definitive answer to the handwashing problem. In reality it would very much depend on the situation, the intensity of the message, and the availability of handwashing materials (e.g., the United States vs. Sudan). It does give us a baseline from which to begin changing our R_0 depending on what actions the players take, how much effort they put into their campaign, and how dire the circumstances are.

Disease parameters

The SIR model is how the disease will end up, but not where epidemiology starts. Most epidemiological investigations start with a cluster of disease that will lead to an eventual outbreak. While we care about bulk transmission and statistics during the epidemic's spread phase, during the initial phase of the disease epidemiologists will be tracing out individual cases, identifying contacts, and determining the basic parameters for the disease (which they will then use in their models). This involves essentially unrolling the components of R_0 so that we can understand in detail how the disease behaves.

We care about the following characteristics of the disease:

- *Susceptibility.* This is an epidemiological term meaning the proportion of the population that can be infected by the disease. Here we mean it in its clinical sense: when an individual is exposed to a disease what is the chance that they will develop symptoms. Susceptibility in a population will vary according to many different factors including microbiome, sex, temperature, environment, age, chance, history, immunity, nutrition, and genetics.[177] This is an important factor to understand in game design, because even if people are exposed, some of them won't develop clinical symptoms while others will.

- *Transmissibility.* What mechanisms does the disease use to infect individuals? Diseases that infect individuals from other infected people are contagious diseases. Transmission routes can be divided into:

  o *Vectors.* Some diseases, like malaria or Zika, are transmitted by animal or insect vectors.

  o *Aerosols.* Aerosols typically come from someone coughing or sneezing, but they can also come from physical items such as envelopes. Aerosols can be large (droplets) or small (particles) depending on the disease and the infectivity. The breakpoint between droplets is usually the Brownian size of 1-5 microns (μm), which will stay suspended due to Brownian motion. Things that stay suspended in the air column can travel a lot farther than bulk liquid droplets, but they are susceptible to environmental factors such as dilution, UV light, and humidity.

  o *Sexual contact.* Sexually transmitted diseases (STD) are another form of vector, even for diseases you might not immediately associate with STD, such as COVID-19.[178]

  o *Fomites.* Fomite refers to any physical object that might be infectious, such as doorknobs, bedding, clothing, etc. Fomite transfer can also be called vehicle-borne transmission.

- *Incubation period.* Or how long the delay is between infection and beginning to show symptoms. The incubation period can depend on both the susceptibility of the victim as well as the degree of exposure.

- *Latency.* The time between when the person gets the disease and when they become infectious.

- *Symptomatic period.* This is the time between when a person begins to show symptoms and they stop showing symptoms. That can occur because the person recovers, dies, or the disease goes dormant.

---

[176] Judah, G. et al. (2009) "Experimental Pretesting of Hand-Washing Interventions in a Natural Setting," *American Journal of Public Health.* 99:S2:S405-S411.

[177] Casadevall, A. and Liise-anne Pirofski. (Jan 2018) What Is a Host? Attributes of Individual Susceptibility," *Infection and Immunity*, 86 (2) e00636-17; DOI: 10.1128/IAI.00636-17

[178] Song, C. et al. (2020) Detection of 2019 novel coronavirus in semen and testicular biopsy specimen of COVID-19 patients medRxiv 2020.03.31.20042333; doi: https://doi.org/10.1101/2020.03.31.20042333 PREPRINT

- *Contagious period.* This can occur when the person becomes infected, or sometime after infection. It can occur before symptoms begin, or only after symptoms are showing. If the individual can spread the disease without showing symptoms it is termed asymptomatic infection. For some diseases the period during which an individual is capable of spreading the disease but is also mobile is a very short period of time. For example, with pneumonic plague patients spread it through aerosol droplets, but they will be mobile and coughing for only a day or so in most cases. After that they will be clearly sick and immobilized. This can represent a significant break on the spread of a disease.

These are a lot of parameters. We can argue that each of these parameters affects the overall transmissibility of the disease. For example, if the contagious period is long, with a long asymptomatic period where individuals are contagious then the disease will spread more easily than a disease which removes the individual almost as soon as they acquire the disease. This can severely limit the spread of a disease, even one that is highly infectious and easily transmitted.

Take, for example, pneumonic plague. For an inhalational exposure the time to first symptoms in primates and humans is typically 2-4 days.[179] Without intravenous antibiotic treatment (post-symptomatic) the time till death is usually another 2-4 days.[180] Given that during the 2-4 day symptomatic period the victim is not feeling terribly well (fever, cough, pneumonia, and gastro-intestinal symptoms) they are not going to be going out and encountering large numbers of the public. In addition, they don't have a lot of time to engage with other people before they become fatalities. This will decrease the overall exposure for each case, even if they are not recognized and isolated. This will mean that the overall R_0 for the disease will be relatively low, depending on the circumstances.

The challenge for game designers is that we are caught in the middle between clinicians and epidemiologists. The clinicians care about data on individuals, their symptoms, treatment, and disease progression. Epidemiologists care about populations, what the time interval between one infection and the next is (generation interval) or the number of cases generated by each case (R_0). Clinicians talk in terms of the disease; epidemiologists talk in terms of populations. What we as game designers most often care about are the particulars of the environment. And the way in which the disease moves around in the environment. This, as we saw during the early days of both the 2001 anthrax event and the COVID-19 response, are not something that either clinicians or epidemiologists have focused on in the past.[181]

It can be difficult getting specific data for a specific disease. Let's take smallpox as an example. The R_0 for smallpox worldwide is approximately 5 (so we need 80% ($P_{herd} = 1 - 1/R_0$) of the population to be immune to develop herd immunity).[182] This can help with epidemiological models, but what if we have a gentleman who is found in a Universities' student center passed out. A few hours after being found he dies. Differential diagnosis immediately suggested a pox virus, and lab results from the CDC confirm smallpox. What do we assume about transmission?

Smallpox is highly infectious through the nasal/oral routes with only a few viral particles being sufficient for infection. The incubation period is 12-17 days.[183] Remember that everything here is a distribution, some take less time while others take longer. The range is given as 7-17 days. The rash forms within 1-2 days while at the onset the individual has high fever, aches, and is often incapacitated. Infectivity begins around day 14 after infection and is highest from days 15 through 19 (for a day 12 onset of symptoms). Infectivity then diminishes until day 26 when it disappears. It is also highly transmissible, one person, isolated in a hospital room with a cough infected 3 floors of a hospital.[184] Vaccination within 4 days of exposure has been shown to provide some immunity.[185]

---

[179] Inglesby, T. et al. (3 May 2000) "Plague as a Biological Weapon," *JAMA* 283:17: 2281-2290.

[180] Inglesby (2000).

[181] During this period of pandemic COVID there is a large number of studies, and even more discussion, about issues of transmission, susceptibility, and fate in the environment. However, many of these factors are still unknown, even for a disease with as much focus as COVID-19.

[182] Brauer (2008).

[183] There are a lot of references on smallpox. The one I'm using here is Henderson, DA., et al. [9 Jun 1999] "Smallpox as a Biological Weapon," *JAMA.* 281:22:2127-2137. You will get a variety of values for the numbers I cite depending on the reference.

[184] Wehrle, P F et al. (1970) "An airborne outbreak of smallpox in a German hospital and its significance with respect to other recent outbreaks in Europe." *Bulletin of the World Health Organization* 43:5:669-79.

[185] Henderson (1999).

So, what does all this mean for our individual sitting in the student center? First, we have to establish a timeline for when the individual was exposed to and contracted the disease. While there won't be a note on him saying when it was, you can bet the players can do the math and figure out when exposure occurred. It will be highly relevant for the law enforcement portion of the game.

Based on the paper we are using for our information; infectivity becomes greatest about 3 days after the onset of symptoms. At this point the individual will have developed pustules and will likely be feeling pretty ill from fever and other symptoms. The individual will have felt bad for the past 3 days prior to becoming highly infectious. We will also need to have the individual do something to spray the disease around, just sitting there won't likely do it. Perhaps allergies or some reason to cough will help us along. Or vomiting is a symptom associated with smallpox, but that will draw a lot of attention and response and likely minimize the number of people exposed. The good news is that just one hearty sneeze should do enough damage, given the infectivity of the virus, to present a threat to the entire population in or moving through the student center.

But let's look at the sneeze in detail (sorry about this). First the sneeze will produce a distribution of droplets, which we can assume all contain some concentration of virus. However, a lot of that sneeze will fall to the floor within a 3-18 foot radius of the individual, assuming recent studies related to COVID are to be believed.[186] Some of the exhaled particles may be in the magic range of 1-5 microns, which will linger in the air but also be big enough not to be exhaled easily out of the lungs when breathing. This range is ideal for agents to travel long distances but still be infectious. However, as the sneeze propagates outward it will dilute, as will the microparticles that accompany it. This will decrease the concentration of the virus until eventually you get less than an infectious dose, or at least a low probability of getting infected from the dose. Another factor will be the rate of passage of the individuals in the room. Students moving quickly through the area will have less total exposure to the virus than an individual sitting next to the person. All of these factors come into play when considering what the exposed population looks like in your game. And players, especially medical or epi players, will notice unless you have a good story to back up your results.

It will also affect the first responders, as well as the hospital personnel in the emergency room. At least until they do a differential diagnosis. If the emergency room is backed up there is an additional population that could be infected. Not to mention the EMS in the ambulance, and any other first responders involved. If he is suspected of a crime and sent to an institution like a jail prior to diagnosis, that in turn will generate another possible population.[187]

This suggests it can take time to start and epidemic from just one isolated event. Disease outbreaks take time and can go unnoticed for weeks or months.[188] Virulent diseases like smallpox often have such debilitating symptoms that the victim is not ambulatory when most infectious. However, once we infect a sufficient number of people in the student center, and the hospital, it can become difficult to trace, isolate, and vaccinate everyone exposed, allowing the general epidemiological models (and the impressively high R_0 of 5) to take over. It is likely that modern medical equipment, a massive federal and state response, and effective public health measures would greatly reduce the rate of transmission in our case. But that would be up to the players.

---

[186] And there are a lot of papers suddenly coming out on these topics. For example: Dhand, R. and J. Li (16 Jun 2020) Coughs and Sneezes: Their Role iN transmission of Respiratory Viral Infections, Including SARS-CoV-2," *AJRCCM* in press. 10.1164/rccm.202004-1263PP; Pendar, M. and J. Pascola (2020) "Numerical modeling of the distribution of virus carrying saliva droplets during sneeze and cough," *Physics of Fluids*, 32 https://doi.org/10.1063/5.0018432; Shafaghi, A. et al. (16 Jul 2020) "On the Effect of the Respiratory Droplet Generation Condition on COVID-19 Transmission," *Fluids*, 5:113: doi:10.3390/fluids5030113

[187] Wehrle (1970) will be very helpful if that happens.

[188] For example, in the case of SARS-CoV-2 there may have a period of "cryptic spread" in China where the virus mutated away from its animal origins, going undetected until a cluster of pneumonias occurred. Zhang, Y. and E. Holmes (16 Apr 2020) "A Genomic Perspective on the Origin and Emergency of SARS-CoV-2," *Cell*, 181:223-227. And Du, Z. et al. (2020) "Using the COVID-19 to influenza ratio to estimate early pandemic spread in Wuhan, China and Seattle, US," *EClinicalMedicine*, https://doi.org/10.1016/j.eclinm.2020.100479

Chapter 10: Chronic and non-infectious diseases

Not all diseases are transmissible, and the vast majority of things that epidemiologists and public health professionals worry about fall into the broad range of chronic diseases. These include things like cancer, heart disease, diabetes, addition, and mental health issues. Chronic and other non-transmissible diseases can present issues for game designers because:

- The underlying cause and effect are poorly understood and often based on statistical, as opposed to biological, relationships.
- Patient behaviors can play a significant role in many of these diseases.
- Because behavior matters public information and communication, including getting populations to adopt various behaviors and practices, can be part of the overall public health response to these diseases.

It is not common to do games on these types of disease. This is perhaps because they do not present as an urgent or immediate problem, and don't generally involve law enforcement or other security issues. At the same time, they can present us some of the more interesting challenges as we think about information, populations, and statistical models in our designs.

Statistical analysis

Epidemiologists are not all about infectious disease progression through populations. They also collect data and try to understand the frequency, causes, and other associations of disease within society. These can be chronic diseases, or diseases associated with behaviors or environmental factors. In many ways these diseases are more difficult to analyze than the typical infectious disease. You don't have a microorganism to identify, understand, and track. Instead, you often have many different things that could impact the progress of the disease, many of which are difficult to isolate as individual factors. The causes are intertwined in the data, and in the real world. It can be difficult to figure out which are the most important, have the most clinical impact, and how all of the different factors are related to each other.

When developing games associated with chronic or non-epidemic diseases, you will need to understand both the human and medical factors that affect the progress of the disease. You don't necessarily have to do detailed statistics on the disease, often the actual epidemiologists and medical professionals have a hard time doing that, rather you need to understand the relationships between variables, and how the variables may change based on interventions. This will allow you to project the results of player actions on the disease progress, just as you would for any other disease. The projections may not be accurate, but if they are based on analog or historical data, they will at least seem realistic enough for the players to accept and the game to proceed.

For example, in the case of a game on vaping you might need to understand the relationship between the economic aspects (cost, marketing, sales, availability) and the perception amongst various demographic groups of the safety and desirability of vaping. If players decided to implement taxes to increase cost, then you would need to decide how much that would drive down demand given all the other factors.

To do this you will often need to:

- *Relate medical interventions to disease prevention and outcomes.* If there is a new test that is developed to determine if someone has the potential for cancer, then that may reduce the incidence of disease by a certain amount if there is a potential intervention. You will need to be able to project that reduction based on the type of intervention. This is an intensely medical question and can be difficult to adjudicate in advance because you never know what the players will suggest or do. A couple of techniques that can help:

    o *Use a doctor.* Medical professionals know a lot about prevention and outcomes. They can become your walking database. Even if they are only players, pulling them aside and asking for their help usually works.

    o *Read the literature.* Most treatments have a timeline from initial detection to deployment. In addition, they have a certain success rate as they move through the system. You can use this data for the disease you are working on to gauge an approximate value for your players' treatment. After all, if it doesn't exist the actual data for its success does not exist either.

- *Incorporate non-medical interventions into disease progress.* Mayor Bloomberg's restriction on drink sizes in New York City in 2012 is an example of a non-medical intervention designed to lower incidence of disease.[189] Information operations such as a marketing campaign would also fall into this category. These can be difficult to assess, but polling data and medical studies of different types of interventions are a place to start. For example, on the soda ban you can find references providing different types of policies[190] than can reduce soda consumption, and if you prefer a tax solution then a review study found that it was reasonably predictive of weight loss in populations.[191]

- *Link interventions to costs.* Most interventions will impose some cost on either the population, the government, or the medical system. Costs may be non-monetary—in the case of the drink ban the cost was to the population's ability to purchase the size drinks they wanted. Calculating what the exact cost of an intervention is, and the potential political and social fallout, will need to rely on numbers provided by either subject matter experts, past experience, or the players themselves. The easiest calculation is the cost of an existing medicine, you just look it up. However, the cost of a new or reformulated medicine, one that has never been seen before and was developed in the game, will need to draw on analogs.

- *Project the impact of the social trajectory of the disease.* Some diseases don't cross the threshold into public discourse: hantavirus, for example.[192] Others like Zika[193] and Ebola[194] capture considerable attention. Surprisingly, there has been considerable work done on relating the media environment and attention on disease to the overall disease response. We will discuss this more when in the section on information operations.

None of these studies, papers, or references are either perfectly matched to what we need to do, nor are they somehow definitive and exact predictors of the factors we need to predict. But in all cases, they give us more evidence than we had before we used them, and they also give us an idea of what the correct trend in the data is. If, for example, the study on the effect of taxes on weight loss had found a counter-intuitive result, that weight had gone up, for example, then we would have an interesting trend that we could include in our game, with at least some referral point as to cause and effect if we were challenged. Throughout this book we are referring to using studies and data to inform our gaming choices, but in reality, it is a wholistic and approximate program that gains both credibility and accuracy from use of primary sources.

As an example, lets discuss a game on preventing and responding to a significant outbreak of heart disease in women. The objective is to understand issues surrounding women's health, heart disease, and heart disease treatment and prevention in rural, economically challenged, areas with limited access to health care. What actions should HHS take? The Office of the Assistant Secretary for Health has been tasked to lead a task force finding solutions for this problem. The task force will include CDC, SAMHSA, Agency for Healthcare Research and Quality (AHRQ), FDA, Centers for Medicare and Medicaid Services (CMS), Indian Health Service (IHS), and Office of Assistant Secretary for Public Affairs (ASPA).[195]

We are going to do a large-scale seminar game, with 30-40 representatives from all of the concerned agencies. The origin of the problem will be media reporting of local health and public health officials which drives the White House to become involved and direct HHS to initiate a program to solve the problem. So, the question for the group is: what is the problem, and how will they address it?[196]

---

[189] Kobler, J. (12 Jun 2013) "Study: NY Soda Ban Would Be Effective," *US News and World Report.* https://www.theguardian.com/us-news/2020/jan/14/man-requests-sword-fight-ex-wife-lawyer-settle-legal-dispute

[190] Muth, N. et al. (Apr 2019) "Public Policies to Reduce Sugary Drink Consumption in Children and Adolescents," Pediatrics. 143:4

[191] Backholer, K. et al. (Apr 2016) "The impact of a tax on sugar-sweetened beverages according to socio-economic position: a systematic review of evidence," *Public Health Nutrition.* doi:10.1017/S136898001600104X

[192] Douglass, R. et al. (15 Jul 2015) "State-by-State Incidences of Hantavirus Pulmonary Syndrome in the United States, 1993-2004," *Vector-Borne and Zoonotic Diseases.* 5:2:189-192.

[193] Tizzoni, M, et al. (12 Mar 2020) "The impact of news exposure on collective attention in the United States during the 2016 Zika epidemic," *PLoS Computational Biology.* 16:3: e1007633. https://doi.org/10.1371/journal.pcbi.100763

[194] Sell, T. et al. (Jan 2017) "Media Messages and Perception of Risk for Ebola Virus Infection, United States," *Emerging Infectious Diseases.* 23:1:108-111.

[195] In reality many more agencies and departments might be involved, we can just consider these for simplicity.

[196] We won't let them simply define the problem as a public information one, though public information will be one component of the overall problem.

We can quickly find studies involving identifying risk factors for heart disease in rural women.[197] In the study nursing intervention in addition to community interventions significantly improved things like intake of fruit, total fruit and vegetable intake, and increased willingness to eat fruits and vegetables. But it is likely that nursing interventions for an entire population will be expensive, and in some areas like the one we are concerned with there may not be enough nurses. Players may then look to other areas, like determining where and in what populations the incidence is occurring. If it were in nursing homes, for example, targeted interventions there may be required. But who is responsible within HHS for nursing homes, and what capabilities and capacities do they have?

In preparing for the game, we will need to consider all of the various directions the players may go. We will need to prepare the ground truth that we will present to the players through media, studies, and medical community reporting. For example, we may decide that those living in extremely isolated areas have increased stress due to lack of employment opportunities and loss of medical, food, and other support services. These particular populations are stressed and placing stress on the few urban hospitals in the area. Specific presentations of the disease may occur because the individuals frequently drink well water and can only eat shelf stable food due to frequent power losses. They may also have difficulty getting to primary or secondary treatment, increasing mortality.

Part of the challenge the players will face is simply figuring out what is going on, then addressing it. Studies and research will take time so we can expect our game to have large steps in game time. During these steps the White House may not be happy with the rate of progress on the issue and media coverage will continue. This may force players to act before they really know what is going on. No matter what the players do there will be consequences. Should they decide to intervene with policies and lifestyle modifications then there may be political issues raised. If they intervene with medical and hardware solutions then the cost may increase. The role of the state in these interventions will need to be represented, as will the local medical, hospital, and public-health systems.

The best result for the game would be a discussion between the researchers, public health professionals, hospitals, medical professionals, and HHS leadership about the cost and opportunities for intervention and different strategies that might be politically and economically practical. It would also highlight the various equities of the organizations involved along with possible capabilities that they had to address this issue. The groups would also get the chance to meet each other and work together on a high visibility problem before the event actually occurred.

We will describe a sample game on this topic in greater detail in the next section.

Chronic and non-infectious disease

In the previous sections we discussed diseases that were acute, or moved through the cycle of infection, symptoms, transmission, and recovery. There are also diseases that are either non-infectious or become chronic as opposed to acute. Chronic diseases generally last a year or more and have some sort of long-term impact on those affected. Chronic disease may be either transmissible or non-transmissible and for our purposes can include environmental factors such as chemical poisoning. Throughout this paper, including here, we exclude any radiological hazards either in the environment or through deliberate exposure.

AIDs is an example of a disease that is both transmissible and is chronic in that there is no current cure. Patients don't recover, they continue to survive with the disease. Heart disease is an example of a disease that is not transmissible, but one that occurs through genetic, lifestyle, and other factors. Mercury poisoning is an example of an environmental factor that produces chronic outcomes. It's not a disease per-se but causes a medical situation that resembles a disease. Our example in the section on research and statistics in epidemiology was for an outbreak of heart disease. Games on these types of disease are uncommon because they don't have the immediate response and decision focus of acute disease. But they may be just as important for allocating resources and coordinating medical strategies.

As we saw in the example on heart disease in women you may need to understand the disease epidemiology in order to develop a scenario. The causes of the disease can be complex, multi-variate and not well understood.

---

[197] Fahs, Pamela Stewart et al. (2013) "Promoting heart health in rural women." *The Journal of rural health : official journal of the American Rural Health Association and the National Rural Health Care Association* vol. 29:3: 248-57. doi:10.1111/j.1748-0361.2012.00442.x

For example, in heart disease the relative contribution of genetics, environmental, health, age, and other factors are known, but not accurately parameterized. We know, for example, that exercise cuts heart disease and can tie that to amount and demographics.[198]

The primary things to consider when building a game on chronic disease include:

- *Cost.* Chronic diseases usually have high costs to both the patient, health care system, and governmental programs. Preventative and treatment measures are often high cost and can endure for a long time. For diabetes the direct cost of treatment is approximately $10,000 in additional per year medical costs for individuals. Most (67%) of that cost is to government programs. Indirect costs include cost at work and lost productive capacity.[199] Games on chronic disease will often weigh cost vs. risk in ways that games on more acute disease response will not.

- *Public information.* Many chronic diseases are related to social, economic, or group conditions. These can be politically charged when related to disease and disease outcomes. The current political situation in many countries only increases the potential for these diseases to become politically polarized. This can create a tricky set of public-information and social-action decisions for government players in a game on disease response. The decision by Mayor Bloomberg of New York City to ban certain size beverage cups is an example of a public health decision that provoked a popular response.[200]

- *Communications, coordination, and cooperation.* Coordination that has to happen in acute response operations is urgent, and imperative. That cuts through a lot of the normal impediments to cooperation and coordination, which occur in the day-to-day execution of a department's mission. But chronic-response operations take time. Sometimes years, and often there is no end in sight. They are part of the normal workday mission of those involved. This means that all of the rivalries, hostilities, competitions, and agendas that impede communications, coordination and cooperation in normal times applies in these games.

The challenge for chronic games is to build scenarios that bring out the challenges associated with information, cooperation, and cost. Cost and information can be difficult to bring out in games.

Cost is challenging to include because of the detail and introspection that is required to manage cost processes. If players are focused on spreadsheets, they won't be interacting with each other or the game. One option is to abstract that cost element in the games. Instead of a detailed budget each group has a virtual budget of coins, cubes, or other materials that they can allocate as part of a budget process. Detail will be removed so you won't be allocating for salaries, utilities, services, and loan payments for a hospital, you will just be allocating the rolled-up cost for the hospital. Keeping cost in big increments is a tool frequently used in hobby games as it is far more manageable that complex calculations.

When you roll up cost players can (and often do) object. Players can sometimes be literal minded and not be able to abstract away detail the way most gamers can. "But I want to cut the cost of the linen services to pay for it, and I would be able to…" can be irritating for players and controllers alike.

The behavioral aspects of disease are even harder to account for. How much does a public relations campaign focused on getting people to change their behavior actually result in changed behavior? Note that this is a campaign by the players directed at the affected population, not competing political messages directed at other populations, like voters. It depends on a variety of confounding variables, and, based on current experiences with COVID-19 can either result in some benefit, or actually backfire. Continuing with the example of heart disease, you as the game designer will know that it will come up as an option for the players during the game, so you can do some research on potential outcomes. The actual effects will depend on the population, the message, and the type of behavior being targeted.[201] For example in Cavill (2004), the meta-analysis shows an

---

[198] Francis, K. (May 1996) "Physical Activity in the Prevention of Cardiovascular Disease," *Physical Therapy*, 76:5;456-468

[199] https://www.diabetes.org/resources/statistics/cost-diabetes

[200] "Mayor Bloomberg's proposed extra-large soda ban combines the draconian government overreach people love; with the probable lack of results they expect." – Jon Stewart (see, http://www.cc.com/video-clips/wdlzd8/the-daily-show-with-jon-stewart-drink-different)

[201] See, for example, Wakefield, Melanie A et al. (2010) "Use of mass media campaigns to change health behaviour," *Lancet (London, England)* vol. 376,9748 : 1261-71. doi:10.1016/S0140-6736(10)60809-4 and Cavill, N. and A. Bauman. (2004) "Changing the way people think about health-enhancing physical activity: do mass media campaigns have a role?" *Journal of sports sciences* vol. 22,8: 771-90. doi:10.1080/02640410410001712467

11% reduction in heart disease following a "well designed" media campaign. This, and the variation given in the same article, could be used to assess player media campaigns in a game setting. If you went back to the original sources (Cavill, 2004) is a review article) you could create a table of message, coverage, target demographic, and outcome that would allow you to interpolate between the different choices that the players might make with their campaigns.

Chapter 11: Information, cyber, and politics

In addition to the practical effects of the disease there are some other factors to consider when designing disease-response games. Most of the non-tactical elements of disease response involve providing public information in order to influence behaviors. In an epidemic this may involve information designed to slow the spread of a disease. For chronic diseases this may be information about changes in behavior that will reduce incidence of the disease. This public signaling can become entangled with many other types of information operations, including cyber operations and public affairs.

Information operations (IO) refer to all forms of manipulation of information. Here we distinguish information operations from cyber, though US joint doctrine does not. [202] This can be positive, such as governments providing accurate information designed it influence behavior. On the other hand, information operations can be used to disrupt the public health response through the deliberate dissemination of incorrect information. Operations of the Russian Internet Research Agency are a current example of such operations. [203] Cyber-attacks against medical systems can also be part of a disease response scenario.

While in this book we are focused on disease response, we also want to touch on issues of information operations that matter for disease response games. Disease response has several information touchpoints that will affect your games.

Public information, public affairs, and the media.

How the players manage their relationship with the press will be an important factor in most disease-response games. Politicians often want to downplay the severity of a disease in order to prevent panic; medical personnel want to get information out on how to minimize the spread of a disease; and, in some cases, there may be legal or moral imperatives to release certain information. The interplay of all these factors can become a game in itself. It is difficult to simulate media play in games because professional players often discount its role unless they have senior-level government or political experience. It can also be challenging for game control to generate sufficient media feeds like those that would be occurring in an actual response.

There are several ways in which media can be incorporated into games:

- *The scenarist approach:* In this approach the media are the backdrop for how information is presented to players. The designers work with a studio and actors to create short video news reports (or in some cases print editions) that convey what is happening in the game world to the players. This technique is often used in strategic, high visibility, games that have an element of showmanship associated with them. The down-side to using video in games is that it can be expensive to hire actors and a studio, and the video script will lock scenario elements in well before the game design is finished. It can also be hard to adjust the video reporting to take into account player actions.

- *Media as part of control:* Again, as with the scenarist approach the media simply become another way to present information to the players. Control tells the players what is going on in the media either directly, or through simulated news summaries, usually print. The advantage over the previous approach is that this is far cheaper, and controllers can dynamically adjust the news to reflect the situation. The downside is that it is far less believable and can have less impact on players. Impact on players can be increased by using metrics such as polling numbers or voting. This works best if rival political parties are simulated in the game, with power changing hands in an "election" that is based on media and public parameters.

- *Media players:* In this case reporters are brought in to simulate the media. This has the advantage of providing an adaptable media presentation that has enormous credibility with the players. The downside is that you have to include media representatives in your games which may affect game play and willingness to share information by the players. Media representatives can often also devolve into

---

[202] We are distinguishing cyber from IO to emphasize the differences between the techniques used to account for them in games. In joint US doctrine cyber is a component of information operations. Joint doctrine essentially defines information operations as a kitchen sink of items only related in that they somehow affect information. Joint Chiefs of Staff (9 Oct 1998) *Joint Doctrine for Information Operations*.

[203] Howard, P. et al. (2018) The IRA, Social Media and Political Polarization in the United States, 2012-2018.

observer or subject-matter expert mode, in which they lecture the players on media issues as opposed to play their role in the game.

- *Have players represent the media:* This is similar to bringing in media players, but it circumvents the problem of having players reluctant to share with actual media. At the same time the capabilities and experience levels of the players representing the media will mean that you often get only a caricature of the actual media. It also means that some players with skills relevant to the problem will be representing media instead of their original task.

There are no perfect solutions to the problem of representing media in games. If actual media professionals are available and can be used in the game then that produces the greatest credibility and most realistic media play. However even with professional media players the full spectrum of the modern media, from Facebook to blogs to mainstream media will not be simulated. It is the complex interaction of all these media sources that produces the overall media environment for decision-makers. This is the advantage of control's managing media play: different points of view can be brought in and emphasized to the players as decisions get made.

The key is to ask which interest groups and political points of view might be affected by the decisions of each player. This can be challenging because medical decisions are often ambiguously intertwined with social and political points of view. When we think of warfighting, we have some basis to estimate how the public—or at least certain political factions within the public—will respond to various provocations. Medical decisions can be more complex.

In the case of COVID-19 there is the disparity between different races in infection rate.[204] This has had an impact on the overall political conversation and could affect how treatments and vaccine rollouts are perceived. It bridges the disease epidemiology with political and social factors.[205] Incorporating issues like this into a game will raise the social stakes for anyone participating in the game and require control to decide the effects of player actions on media and political discourse.

Any inter- or intra-group effects from the disease used in the game should be viewed as a potential media or political issue that can challenge player actions. For example, if a vaccine or treatment for an otherwise untreatable disease were to be found in one country, the allocation of the item might become subject to international political considerations as well as issues of equity and privilege between developed and less-developed countries. If this suddenly intersects national security concerns the problem becomes even more complicated.

Sorting these issues out in the real world is difficult, sorting them out in games is equally difficult and can dominate players' time and discussions.

Cyber actions

Cyber actions can become integrated with disease response if the nature of the response triggers conflict or integrates into an ongoing conflict. It can also represent a potentially lucrative opportunity for those in the ransomware or malware business. Even if there are no actors with intent on exploiting the disease response, coincidental events, such as a ransomware attack on a hospital system, can exacerbate the overall difficulty of the response. It is also likely that the need for urgent action within the context of the response creates its own set of vulnerabilities and increases the attack surface available to bad actors.

In the current COVID-19 response (2020/21) there are reports that cyber actors may be targeting digital systems, information, and networks associated with vaccine production.[206] Cyber activity may occur for any number of reasons, and, if it affects the ability to respond to a disease, may present a significant challenge to players. If nation states are the originator of the cyber action then it could be to protect or expand their ability to fight the disease. You could postulate that cyber actors in a game would attempt to obtain data or information on vaccines or treatments so as to allow their national production capabilities to ramp up production at the same rate as those developing the treatment. Or you could envision that a nation state might try to impede development if it had an advantage economically or militarily that it would lose should treatments or vaccines become available.

---

[204] https://www.cdc.gov/coronavirus/2019-ncov/need-extra-precautions/racial-ethnic-minorities.html

[205] https://www.americanprogress.org/press/statement/2020/04/30/484337/statement-caps-neera-tanden-applauds-introduction-covid-19-racial-ethnic-disparities-task-force-act/

[206] Sanger, D. and Nicole Periroth. (13 May 2020) "U.S. to Accuse China of Trying to Hack Vaccine Data, as Virus Redirects Cyberattacks," *New York Times.* https://nyti.ms/3cniK6u

Non-nation state actors could also become involved, whether simply to disrupt the response for terroristic reasons or to engage in criminal activity. The ability to distinguish between nation state and sophisticated non-nation state actors also creates a strategic dilemma in the game of attribution and response.

These considerations are most important in strategic level games where all elements of national power are included in the game play. If the effects of a cyber-attack are suddenly magnified by the presence of a disease outbreak, does that justify a more aggressive retaliation posture on the part of the national authorities? If a civilian critical-response system is determined to be vulnerable who is responsible for mandating fixing it? Who pays to secure it? What are the relative roles of the commercial and private sectors in a medical situation? Questions like these can easily occupy legal and political players in a large strategic disease-response game in which there is a significant national security element.

You can include cyber actions in your game through:

- *Cyber players.* In this case you have players representing the cyber actors or groups in the game. If they are part of a nation-state team in the game then they get their objectives from their team. If they are not directly associated with a nation state, or the nation is not represented by players, then control determines their objectives. The cyber players have to propose ways to use cyber accomplish their objectives. This sort of structure works well when you have creative players who know something about enterprise level cyber. Without the player having cyber knowledge you risk the players being unable to develop realistic actions and capabilities. Often what happens is either the player who lacks understanding does not play cyber, or weakly goes through the motions because they are confused. If you simply give the players their targets, objectives, and tools you might as well have them as part of control as they have little or no agency [207]in the game.

- *Control injects.* In this case control is in charge of cyber play and has already developed various attacks and events that will occur in the game. This is well suited to operational or tactical games where medical and disaster-response players have little or no ability to affect the overall course of cyber events. If their hospital computers go down due to a ransomware attack then they call someone to fix them and adjust. If data for a series of experiments is corrupted then they have to adjust their protocols or delay rollout. Actions beyond the scope of the game such as defense, retaliation, or attribution will be done by law enforcement or national authorities outside of the game, as represented by control.

- *Menu of options.* For operational level games involving the interagency process it will be possible for different agencies to respond to cyber events. But they will not be able to dynamically adjust their capabilities within the timeframe of most disease response operations. They are stuck with essentially what they have in terms of cyber capabilities when the game begins. This leads to the idea of a "cyber menu" or "cyber cards" where capabilities are presented to the players as fixed options, with some variation, that they can choose to execute if they wish. This could include everything from the ability to deploy defensive teams to shore up systems,[208] to the ability to enter and exploit, or destroy, adversary systems. Law enforcement capabilities to collect cyber forensics or trace back attacks could also be represented. This technique maintains some control over the capabilities introduced into the game, allows inexperienced players to still "play" cyber, while still giving players agency to affect game outcomes with cyber.

In a large-scale disease response cyber will provide friction and challenges at the national level, as we are seeing with COVID-19. This interaction provides another layer of complexity into game play but requires cyber expertise on the part of both control and the players in order to pull off successfully.

Information operations

We distinguish information operations from cyber operations by the target of the attacks. In information operations a population's understanding, information, or attitudes are the target, while in a cyber-attack digital

---

[207] I use the term "agency" to mean "ability to act." It incorporates both the capability to act, along with the actor's willingness to act, and their perception of their ability to act. Thus it is more than just "can you do something" but also do you believe you can do something. It matters for player engagement in games.

[208] Though this can be difficult due to the diversity of systems and the need for long-term experience for the network defenders. More likely they would issue a contract to a firm that specializes in whatever defensive measures need to be implemented.

information, networks or systems are the target. A cyber-attack could assist or enable information operations, and it is often seen as a component of information operations.

With COVID-19 we are currently seeing how an informationalized environment reacts to a major pandemic response. We have always incorporated information issues in disease-response games, whether it was "miracle cures" that the FDA would have to chase down or misinformation about vaccines or treatments. However, the sheer chaotic breadth and depth of the information flood in today's environment means that previous assumptions need to be expanded.

When designing games on disease response we need to take into account different ways in which information can affect the progress of the response and different populations. We can divide the information into categories according to the degree the information is directed or deliberately generated, and the target of the information:

- *Random, individual.* This is the 'random noise" of rumors and other speculation that will surround a disease outbreak. The idea that vitamin C might cure or prevent the disease. Or that a particular combination of drugs might be effective. There is no malice or self-interest behind these rumors, and they are targeted at treatment of individuals.

- *Deliberate, individual.* These are the inevitable scams and false claims that surround a disease response. Someone claims that they have the cure for the disease if you only send them $19.95.

- *Random, groups.* In this category we place all of the conspiracy theories, internet memes, and other information campaigns directed at groups of people. These are not necessarily directed or built with intention, but they have advocates and individuals within the movement that promote them. Sometimes for personal gain. Examples might be that cell towers cause disease,[209] or that a conspiracy exists where lizard people disguised as scientists are creating the disease.[210]

- *Deliberate, groups.* Organized actors such as nation-states or political groups can also exploit the information environment in order to sow distrust or confusion within a response operation. This is likely to be part of a larger competition between groups, where one group seeks to gain advantage by exploiting the presence of the disease to advance its cause. A nation state that decreases overall compliance with public health measures in a rival country might benefit from the economic or military disruption that occurs due to higher incidence of disease. This quickly becomes an interagency or national security issue.

These types of information disruptors can affect disease response at all levels of game, tactical, operational and strategic. If rumors and innuendo suggest that vaccines may be harmful, fewer members of the susceptible group may show up to get vaccinated. This may require additional or different messaging as part of a tactical operation. Rumors or deliberate mis-information directed at a particular group may require a response rooted in the that group or community. This could require everything from finding translators to building links to community leaders in that group.

Incorporating these types of information operations into games can be done by:

- Assigning the role of the "public" to a player and letting them come up with the public's reactions to player actions. This requires a relatively knowledgeable and creative player to make it work, but when it works it can give a lot of credibility to actions or effects that the other players would otherwise dismiss. This also is a common way of featuring public opinion in matrix games.

- Control actively plays the information environment. Players can issue statements and covertly create rumors, but control adjudicates the outcomes based on the current state of play. This, again, puts the responsibility for open-minded and creative actions on control and works best with an experienced controller who understands all of the various dimensions of the current information environment.

- Scripting information events into the game. Scripted events disassociate game actions from player actions and are a recipe for things going badly in a game. They should be avoided because the intent of both playing information operations and running a game is to react to the player actions, not to run a script against the players. The only cases where this works is games where the players' roles in the

---

[209] https://arstechnica.com/tech-policy/2020/05/prepare-for-cell-tower-attacks-by-5g-covid-19-conspiracy-theorists-us-warns/
[210] https://www.theatlantic.com/national/archive/2013/04/12-million-americans-believe-lizard-people-run-our-country/316706/

game have little or no control over the information environment, which plays out as a backdrop to whatever they are doing. In the case of the vaccination clinic, anti-vaxxer protestors or rumors about the vaccination clinic, can be used to affect clinic operations. Players may respond with a public affairs program, but they are not associated with the underlying causes, or national responses, to the situation.

Political circumstances

Ebola, SARS, AIDS, Zika, and COVID-19 all had significant political impact within the United States during the outbreaks. The impacts may have been different, and their scale may have varied according to the disease's penetration into society, but they were all something at least the interagency had to account for. In the case of COVID-19 we are seeing international political and policy fallout from the disease, especially from recriminations[211] about different approaches depending on the culture, politics, and simply who is in charge of a country.[212]

In the past, games could assume a generic rational-actor model for senior level decision-making within most western countries. By that we mean that neo-conservative, liberal, western-focused, assumptions about the value of international institutions, trade, effective governance, and deterrence were all a baseline set of guides for government action. This is no longer the case as other values, goals, and objectives have come to the forefront of politics. This new diversity of ideas and ways of governing can affect how we structure games, as well as the accuracy of our games.

It has become increasingly difficult to incorporate realistic political points of view within games without alienating players who do not share those political views. This has led to game designers generally ignoring divisive or diverse policies or trends in favor of maintaining the usual assumption of progressive western governance.[213] This allows us to investigate the player actions in a de-politicized environment, but at the expense of a less realistic game.

Unfortunately, this de-politicization of games can lead to unrealistic games that do not take into account the diversity of responses to medical and social situations.

The alternative is to introduce political and policy factors that deviate from the usual assumptions about governance. This will increase the realism for games set in the near future. There is no telling what it will do for the accuracy of games set in the far future. But it will introduce difficult subjects and discussions into play and risk bad behaviors developing amongst the players in the game. These can include irrelevant, but long, discussions, players actively arguing with each other, and players separating from the game and refusing to buy into the scenario. None of these are desirable outcomes in a professional game.

A significant risk is that the play becomes a caricature of the current environment as players go "over the top" with their policies and actions. While this may, in some environments, be realistic, it also limits game results to a very specific set of leaders, time, and place. That would have to be integral to the game objectives in order to make the trade-off between accuracy of game play and the very specific and limited nature of game results.

This is a very hard thing to take into account in modern games. It has not been addressed widely in the gaming literature or professional discourse up to this point. However, it is something that requires more research, thought, and design effort than has so far been put into it.

---

[211] https://www.nytimes.com/2020/05/18/us/coronavirus-updates.html
[212] https://www.nytimes.com/2020/05/15/world/americas/brazil-health-minister-bolsonaro.html
[213] I am using the term "progressive" here to mean the internationalist, forward focused, technology enabled, cooperative style of government based in assumptions about the accuracy of science and the importance of traditional institutions associated with many governments in the past. This is different from the inward-focused, revisionist, skeptical, and uncooperative style of governance triggered in recent years by increased migration and other factors.

Chapter 12: Tactical Melioidosis

Tactical level games focus on the particulars of an individual situation. In military parlance they represent individual battles, with units at the company level and below. For our example we will choose the simple problem of dispensing vaccines and prophylaxis in response to an outbreak of disease. The particulars of why the outbreak occurred will drive how many patients we can expect to treat, what exactly they will be getting for treatment, and where the treatment will occur. And how the state and county health departments will deal with these challenges in the very earliest stages of the event.

In our case the challenge is melioidosis, and the location is Brevard County, Florida. In this case there was a terrorist dissemination of the disease along the roads leading into the Kennedy Space Center (KSC) complex, and along neighborhoods during the evening. It was disseminated in "wet" form, meaning the bacteria in solution was sprayed as a mist. This is highly inefficient and has none of the characteristics of anthrax in terms of downwind hazard area nor persistence. Approximately 500 individuals were affected in the morning near the KSC complex and another 1000 in neighborhood surrounding the town. This is a fairly robust dissemination given the circumstances, environment, and disease. We don't need a lot more than this for the game scenario as we are more concerned about the timing of presentation of cases, and the response, than how they obtained the disease. We are also leaving out a lot of details for obvious reasons.

If this seems a lot like the anthrax attack, just wait. Melioidosis is nothing like anthrax.

We will use the actual laydown of hospitals and outpatient care clinics in the county along with the number of beds and reporting chains.

The disease can be acute, subacute, or chronic (for our purposes). Acute melioidosis has an incubation period of 1-21 days with a mean of 9 days. [214] This is actually good, we can have enough cases hit the system to trigger a response, but with the worst days yet to come. All our disease incidents will be inhalational, which will increase the mortality rate. Patients whose immunity has been compromised will likely present first, again enhancing the ability for us to push the scenario toward an earlier point in the outbreak.

How will the cases present? A breakdown of the clinical features of the disease[215] shows that of the cases presenting with acute form of the disease in Thailand:[216]

- 45% of cases the disease had spread with septicemia (87% mortality without intensive care, 50% mortality with intensive care)

- 42% had localize infection without septicemia (9% mortality)

- 12% of cases it had not spread but had septicemia (17% mortality)

- 0.3% of the cases had transient bacteremia.

The split between acute and chronic was 88% acute, 12% chronic. While this is just one study, and was based in Thailand, it gives us numbers that would be consistent with inhaling a significant dose of the bacteria. Inhalation is associated with acute forms of the disease, higher mortality, and pneumonia.[217]

From a maintenance perspective a large number of the septic patients will need critical care, including renal therapy and other forms of managing organ failure. If there is a timely diagnosis and access to antibiotic therapy the mortality rate should be low.[218]

Treatment requires injected or IV antibiotics for 10-14 days (or longer) followed by oral antibiotics for 12 to 20 weeks.[219] The usual antibiotics, doxycycline and ciprofloxacin are not the preferred treatment, instead IV

---

[214] To continue with the theme of "it is hard to build scenarios from the epidemiological literature" here are some of the values for time from exposure to symptoms: (2 days to years) US Army (1997), (1-21 days, mean 9) Currie (2015)

[215] Currie (2015)

[216] Currie (2015)

[217] Currie (2015)

[218] Currie BJ, Fisher DA, Howard DM, et al. (2000) "Endemic melioidosis in tropical northern Australia: a 10-year prospective study and review of the literature." *Clin Infect Dis.* 31:981–986.

[219] Limmathurotsakul, D. et al. "Chronic melioidosis, relapse and latency." In Ketheesan, Natkunam. (2012) *Melioidosis: A Century of Observation and Research.*

ceftazidime is used. This will likely cause challenges for the players, as it is not a drug commonly stocked in counter-terrorism stockpiles, but is readily available in the health system as a generic.[220] And they will need the IV version of the drug. Use of ceftazidime in a clinical study reduced mortality from 74% to 37%. In another study TMP-SMX was added to the ceftazidime which reduced mortality from 47% to 19% but it was not apparent that TMP-SMX made the difference in mortality. Overall, the randomized controlled trials of IV ceftazidime appear to reduce the overall mortality to between 20 and 35%. Other antibiotics were examined in trials and are available as first or second alternative treatments.[221] The bottom line is that this disease is difficult to treat and even with treatment can have a high mortality rate.

The disease does not go away easily either. 5-25% of patients will re-present with a recurrence after they have been successfully cured. This is after a follow-on therapy of 12-20 weeks of oral antibiotics. The recommended antibiotic treatment is TMP-SMX with or without doxycycline. Again, while doxycycline is a common antibiotic, the primary treatment TMP-SMX, while not uncommon (number 121 most prescribed drug),[222] is not a standard treatment for biological warfare agents. The sourcing of both ceftazidime and TMP-SMX will be an early question for the players, especially since each case needs such an extended regime of treatment.

Because mortality depends on early and effective treatment the timing of the disease dissemination, presentation, diagnosis, and treatment will be important. This is essentially a double fake on the players: it will present as a generic respiratory disease, and then the players may assume it's a standard agent like Anthrax.

The clinical presentation will be all over the map, so no one will immediately go "we've had a terrorist attack by melioidosis" because they recognize the symptoms of inhalational melioidosis. Rather they will notice the increase in frequency of cases presenting to the various clinics and hospitals, with a diagnosis of general respiratory disease. This should trigger alarm bells within public health.

Objective

The game is designed to test coordination between state and local public health, military medical, and civilian hospital and medical systems. The primary question is how the county will coordinate care for one to two thousand patients during a major terrorist event. Secondary objectives include:

- How will the state resource a large quantity of IV antibiotics in response to an event?
- How will the presence of military personnel and military installations affect the overall response?
- Will the commercial hospital system be able to adapt to a sudden increase in patients requiring beds?
- Can the Florida National Guard assist with constructing emergency hospitals, or will federal forces need to supply mobile emergency hospitals?

Note that because this is a tactical game, we are not concerned with what anyone is doing outside of the public-health arena. In fact, we are focused on the hospital system and system capacity to treat the patients. The law enforcement effort, the national effort to manage the stockpile, and the higher-echelon laboratory effort to develop a detailed profile of the disease are not relevant in this game.

A lot of lessons from the COVID-19 pandemic response will be factored into the use of laboratories, testing, and hospital capacity management. However, the unique presentation of this disease, combined with the difficulty of treatment and high mortality rate, should present a challenge for even experienced players.

Players

One of the common questions we face in game design is: What are the players doing at the game? What does the game represent in the game world, and what roles do the players have? In this case we have set up the ideal circumstances for a planning game. If we position the game at the moment that confirmatory tests have come back from the Jacksonville LRN laboratory that this is melioidosis (probably 1 day turnaround if they have the PCR probes), then this can be a game about planning how they are going to deal with potential cases.

---

[220] It was listed by the World Health Organization as an essential medicine: World Health Organization (2019). *World Health Organization model list of essential medicines: 21st list.* hdl:10665/325771. WHO/MVP/EMP/IAU/2019.06..
[221] Limmathurotsakul (2012).
[222] https://clincalc.com/DrugStats/Top300Drugs.aspx

The group of players represents a team brought together by the state and local public-health departments to identify ways in which they can manage patient loads from the probable terrorist release. Given the nature of the disease cases could be coming in for many days or weeks. At the time the players are brought together the terrorists have neither been identified nor caught – so they may be continuing to disseminate it even as the group meets.

In order to keep the game focused we don't want a lot of policy, law enforcement, or security people involved in the game. We mainly want medical personnel and public-health planners. Communications personnel might also be helpful as will those responsible for acquiring and distributing any medicinals.

A roll of players may be:

- Country public-health Department

- Representatives from local critical care clinics.

- Representatives of local fire and emergency services departments.

- Medical representatives for the infectious disease components of local hospitals

- Administrative and staff personnel from local hospitals, including military hospitals at Patrick Air Force Base and any clinics at Cape Canaveral Space Force Station.

    o These individuals should understand the hospital's plan for a major disease outbreak and be capable of talking to space, logistics, and personnel issues.

- Representatives from the state and local public health and diagnostic laboratory network.

    o Representatives should be able to identify what capacity the laboratories have, and what they need, and in what quantity

- Representatives from the Florida National Guard and the Florida Department of Health

- Representatives from the Florida Division of Emergency Management (FDEM)

    o The personnel responsible for acquiring, facilitating, moving, and assisting with distribution of vaccines and/or treatments (in this case antibiotics, both courses)

- Representatives from both the Federal Department of Homeland Security and the Centers for Disease Control and Prevention. These may be local liaison officers assigned to the Florida State government.

- While the game is not designed for law enforcement play, in reality the game organizers would invite representatives of the Brevard FBI satellite office and the County Sheriff's Department. This is both for coordination as well as the likelihood that the Sheriff's Department would be called on to help with hospital and medicinal security.

Game concept

The game will be a tabletop role-playing game with each of the players playing the role of their agency in the overall response. Initial injects will include reporting from the local emergency departments, primary care physicians, and walk-in clinics. It will also have the initial test results from the LRN laboratory and the referral to CDC in Atlanta. Law enforcement (FBI – Tampa) will have already assumed its role as the lead agency in response to an assumed terrorism response, with HHS/Public Health and FEMA/FDEM taking on their roles as assigned by the NRF. This will follow on down to the local level with the local incident management system being informed of the event, leaving it to the players to organize themselves according to their local response plan.

All of the players will need to answer some fundamental questions in the game:

- How are they going to estimate the patient load?

    o Calling the CDC won't help much; they may have to rely on law enforcement or the Defense Threat Reduction Agency (DTRA) (through FEMA) to give them some idea of an initial plume size and/or the likelihood of additional attacks. This is something control should have available to give to the players since it is something that comes from outside the player group.

- Given the patient load is substantial, and the patients require critical care for extended periods, how will they manage the patient load?

- How will they acquire, break down, distribute, and manage the treatment regime? Given that it is a two-phased regime over an extended period, how does this complicate their plan?

- What should their public communications be?

- How will the hospitals manage the costs, get reimbursed, and deal with their normal patient loads?

  o What additional supplies, space, and personnel can they expect to need and where will FEMA/FDEM acquire these? Or are they on their own?

- How will they run diagnostics? Will local hospital laboratories be responsible for diagnosis, in which case they will need the PRC/ELISA probes for Melioidosis if they do not already have them, or will the state laboratories be the primary diagnostic resource? How will laboratory capacity be managed and who will manage it?

They will do this through a series of moves in the game. One way to delineate the moves is to have specific questions associated with the phases in the response. For example, the initial question thrown to the assembled group is to estimate requirements. This means not only estimating the number of initial infected, but also the long-term requirements. It also means translating infected numbers into doses of antibiotic, hospital beds, and other resources. The next question is how, exactly, are they going to manage the local hospital system and distribute patients, and then the final phase is assessing the overall impact on the medical system.

An alternative set of moves would be to follow whatever medical emergency plan they have developed at the state and local level. The challenge is that this is not quite a pandemic, it will not come in predictable phases, and the response will not be national (or international). The pandemic response plan does not quite fit but controllers will need to realize it may be what the players gravitate toward given their recent experience with Coronavirus. A better match may be the state's smallpox response plan which naturally emphasizes contact tracing, isolation, and vaccination. It also emphasizes communications. Not a complete fit as human-to-human transmission is rare.[223] But the overall flow—identifying the affected, delivering treatment, and communicating about the disease—is essentially the same.

As with many disease-response games this is a "one sided" game. The conflict in the game will be between the normal operating posture of the hospitals, which is typically to run with only a few vacant beds, and the need to convert substantial numbers of rooms into critical care facilities. The recent experience with COVID-19 will give the players a template to work from, and this game can represent a chance for the players to test that coordination in a slightly different scenario.

Another significant element of the game will be the clinical presentation of the disease and the treatment of its symptoms. Melioidosis presents in many different ways and requires respiratory and other therapies to manage. Diagnostic and symptom management issues should be integrated into the game. This will mean that control will have to provide a representative spectrum of presentations to the different clinics, and an inventory of different patient requirements. Since this will be early in the event the system will not be overly stressed, but players should quickly get the idea that it may eventually be stressed.

Execution

We are going to assume that this game is more of an "around the table" game than a formal seminar game. A good way to manage this game would be for the players to go off and plan, discuss, and decide what they want to do, then return to the "table" for a facilitated discussion about what, exactly, is going to happen that turn. This has the advantage that everyone gets to participate in discussing the plan, but it also gives players the space to think things through on their own.

We will assume that law enforcement does not show up for this game, leaving that aspect of play for another time.

We will also assume that this is a one-day game to include the post-game hotwash (immediate debrief). Which means we won't have a lot of time for multiple turns. This is not an usual occurrence with one day games. When

---

[223] Kunakorn M, Jayanetra P, Tanphaichitra D. (1991) "Man-to-man transmission of melioidosis." *Lancet*. 337: 1290–1291.

you count for 1 hour up front for introductions and game overview, 1 hour for lunch, you only have six hours to play. Realistically the first turn will take the longest (as the players get established in the game), and you will need at least a half hour for the hotwash. So, if you have an 8-hour day suddenly you are looking at six or fewer hours to actually play the game. In this case we will translate this into a longer first turn, and a shorter third, and final, turn.

Once again, we have professionals playing in the game so only a brief introduction to the situation will be required. Players will also need an introduction to how the game will work. In this example we have chosen to divide the game up into phases: response, relief, and long-term recovery. The response phase will be Turn 1.

Turn 1

During the initial turn players will be responsible for understanding what is happening, identifying and understanding the disease, and building an initial response plan. Aerosol release of melioidosis is neither common nor expected so players will need to first understand what has happened and what the implications are. This will require the county planners and the medical professionals to work together. Initial reports will be scattered across the health care system so the players will need to first build a data collection and case reporting plan. Then, once they understand that this might be a large outbreak, they will need to build a plan for how they will deal with the initial influx of patients. This will require everyone, including the hospital systems, to work together. If military bases have been affected, then the procedures for liaison between the military bases and the community will need to be discussed and reviewed.

During Turn 1 control will have the role of making sure the players address all of the relevant planning topics, and fully react to the situation. During this turn control won't be dropping any more injects or information on the players, rather control will want to make sure that all aspects of the process are addressed.

Turn 2

Turn 2 will be the relief phase. The full caseload will be presented to the players at the beginning of Turn 2 by control. Control will need to account for both player actions, as well as the progress of the disease in the community. Turn 2 will likely occur between days 3 and 5 in the outbreak. At peak case load the hospitals will likely be stressed, and there will be stress on getting treatment and prophylaxis out to the community. The County executives and health department, along with their State and Federal partners, will need to identify requirements given the patient load.

Thus, the primary injects at the beginning of Turn 2 will be the total patient load from the initial presentation. These will need to be divided up and assigned geographically so the initial intake facilities can be identified. If they are clustered in the north of the county then southern hospitals may be able to take the overflow, but someone will need to deal with allocation, transport, and, most importantly, billing.

During turn 2 control will want to emphasize whatever the players have left out or forgotten in their planning from Turn 1. Control will also want to monitor turn 2 planning and ask the right questions to make sure the players are covering all of the possible challenges that they may face. For example, when it comes to transport the fire and EMS player should be able to discuss local transport capacity including the excess capacity over what is routinely required. If they don't, control should be aware and ask.

Turn 3

Turn 3 would usually be termed the "recovery" phase but instead here it could be termed the "chronic" phase. Now that the initial push of cases is over, the problem of chronic melioidosis will become an issue. This will mostly affect the medical system, with the security and emergency management players taking a back seat. Because of this this turn comes at the end, and will likely be rather short. Managing large numbers of chronic cases will place a load on both the medical and the insurance system. How to handle this will be something that the players will need to plan for, if they have not already realized it in turns 1 and 2.

The main challenge for non-medical staff will be the public information challenge. How will they manage the general population that may, or may not, be showing symptoms but may, or may not, come down with this disease in another decade or two. Will they need to contract for some sort of test? What will be the position of the CDC and HHS? Will they try and ignore it? If that is the case control will need to push the game forward several years, when cases begin presenting from chronic disease, to again engage the players with the potential long-term consequences. It may be decided that, in fact, the caseload is manageable given that it is spread out (and not on their watch).

This is an example of a tricky sort of move that sometimes occurs in games. If you set up the parameters correctly, the right information feed regarding public attitudes, the right number of cases, and the correct questions then the players will respond in interesting ways. But if you as control fail to set up and manage the scenario correctly the players can quickly just dismiss the problem and overlook many of the implications that, if they had thought about them, they would in fact care about.

Chapter 13: Strategic, Operational, and Tactical Games

We have discussed how to design games, and how disease response, epidemiology and medical information need to be accounted for in games about public health. These are different ways to approach the complex and multi-sided problem of designing professional games. Another way to think about games is by their *scale*. Scale can mean a lot of things in games. For wargames it refers to the size of the battlespace and how long each move takes. It can also be associated with the military concepts of "tactical, operational, and strategic." This is how we use the term here. Tactical games deal with things of smaller scale, think of a game on laying out and running a vaccination line as an example of a tactical game. Operational games focus on organizations and how they work together, while strategic games focus on broad policy options made at the highest levels of government.

Strategic games often focus on how players will use all elements of national power to achieve some sort of objective.[224] This can also be state or local power, but the strategic level tends to integrate across the interagency. Examples include health-response games that incorporate considerations of military action, or law enforcement, into the play. The most important question is often how health capabilities manage to fit in, and find a voice at the table, amongst all of the louder voices from the military, law enforcement, and emergency response. At this level the political and public communications strategies become important considerations as they will often influence practical decisions.

If strategy focuses on policy the operational level focuses on linking policy to results through campaigns. In the military, campaigns are a series of movements and battles. For medical response, campaigns are how different skills, organizations, and technologies will link together in time and space in order to achieve a public health result. For example, an effort that brings together laboratory networks with hospitals and researchers to better understand and treat (or eradicate) a disease, like smallpox, would be an example of an operational campaign. Operational actions focus on practical actions but also bring together different organizational elements to accomplish those actions.

For the military tactics are the employment and actions of forces in the face of the enemy. The tactical level of war is where individual battles are fought. They involve maneuver and employment of individual weapons systems. Thus, a strategic system, such as the nuclear deterrence force, could engage in a tactical wargame which examined the force's ability to strike enemy targets while absorbing hits from the enemy strategic systems. The system is a strategic system with far reaching effects, but the game on the details of nuclear exchange is still a tactical game. For disease games the tactical level is where the medical system engages with the disease process. This could be a vaccination clinic, a hospital system that is managing caseloads, or the process of developing a treatment for a new disease.

In this section we will examine these categories, discuss what topics they cover, and the players that might be involved. Each level is a bit more diverse than you may think it is. In the process of discussing these different game scales, we will also take the opportunity to bring out game design concepts, tips, and tricks that apply.

Strategic games

Strategic games almost always create a situation during which senior policymakers have to go through a series of decisions. Even if players represent whole countries, their perspective is one of the senior leadership or zeitgeist of the country as they navigate through the scenario.[225]

Focusing on the decisions that players make is one way that you can begin the process of putting your game together. What, exactly, do you expect the players to decide during the game? One consideration is whether these decisions are appropriate for the players in the roles they will be assigned. This involves:

---

[224] For a discussion of what tactical-operational-strategic mean see: Joint Chiefs of Staff (22 Oct 2018) *JP-3 Joint Operations*. https://www.jcs.mil/Doctrine/Joint-Doctrine-Pubs/3-0-Operations-Series/

[225] In strategic games players can either represent individuals within the government, a role-playing game, or form a committee that reflects decisions (based on the assumed zeitgeist of the country) made by the whole of government, a committee game. A debate occurred during the 1950s over which style was best, see, for example: Levine, Robers, Thomas Schelling, and William Jones. (May 2991) *Crisis Games 27 Years Later: Plus C'est Déjà Vu*. RAND Report P-7719.

- *Authority.* Do the players' roles have the authority to make the decision? While an emergency room doctor may have the ability to prescribe medication, they probably won't be able to decide how a new vaccine will be developed.

- *Agency.* Even if the players in their roles have the authority, do they have the ability to execute the decision? In other words, the President has the authority to determine how vaccine research will be conducted, but does he have the knowledge and reputation to decide between one method and another?

- *Player knowledge.* In the previous two cases I was focused on the roles that the players have in the game and whether those roles had authority and agency. Now I'm asking whether the players themselves are knowledgeable and familiar enough with the particular question to make an informed decision. In a game with non-medical players, it is unlikely a vigorous and informed debate about different antibiotic treatments will emerge.

So, can the players make an informed decision, are the roles they are playing empowered to make such a decision, and do those roles have the ability to ensure that their decisions are carried out? For strategic games this can be important. In reality the President, Secretary of Health and Human Services (HHS) and the Centers for Disease Control and Prevention (CDC) director all have different roles to play. They don't make the same decisions, the scope of their authority is limited, and even if they had the authority to make a decision, they may not have the ability to really do so. Strategic games have to take this into account when designing scenarios and building player roles.

During the early phases of an event there are an enormous number of possibilities and you can get more strategic decisions on the table than during the middle and end stages of an event. Setting your scenario early in a disease response is desirable if you want the players to explore a lot of alternative policy issues, while setting it later will focus the players on a few clearly defined questions.

In the case of our melioidosis game the strategic situation is pretty clear. An attack with biological agents against a national space launch complex is very much a strategic level attack. It could be that a nation-state is preparing for war by targeting our space launch capability. This consideration would be a major policy issue for the White House. The attack could also be a terrorist attack, with no relationship to a nation-state. In that case the immediate threat may not be to other space launch systems but to any number of possibly vulnerable targets. If that is the case then the need to protect civilians just got a lot bigger. And this may be some strangely natural outbreak, which means that over-reacting may not be in order.

Should the administration wait? If they wait, then they may be vulnerable. If they act prematurely, they may waste resources protecting the wrong target set. Early in the event these possibilities all seem equally likely and present the administration with a difficult trade-off.

You will also note that these decisions are far different from the decisions that players in the game we describe in Chapter 12 will make. In that case the decisions are all tactical and have little relationship with the decisions that the national leadership will be making. While players (and their real-world counterparts) may want to speculate on what is going on, they will have neither the authority nor ability to influence decisions about terrorists or retaliation. Likewise, the strategic players will decide to deploy the stockpile and whether the event at the Cape warrants being declared a national emergency, but they won't get involved in deciding how the local hospital system operated. At least at first.

Later in the game at least some of the terrorist will have been caught. We can now add that one cell was targeting North American Aerospace Defense Command (NORAD) headquarters at Peterson Air Force Base, Colorado. Law enforcement investigations quickly revealed that they had ties to a foreign power, and intelligence reporting says the foreign power is moving its forces to threaten a partner of the United States. This changes the game completely. Now players at the strategic level are quite focused.[226] This is a game where the disease response is one component of a major national security event. The focus will be on tracking down the rest of the suspected actors, building a case for attribution, and debating about deterrence and response options. Medical will quickly take a back-seat at the strategic level as White House and National Security Council (NSC) players debate about possible retaliation and the consequent escalation.

---

[226] The players at the local level are probably still trying to sort out reimbursement to the hospital system, deal with a major influx of walking well, and navigating a complex political environment where the state and federal agencies all are trying to run their response. But the local agencies still have no influence or authority on the strategic issues in play.

In this example we focused on a national security event. If instead we had a disease event like Zika the timing issue would still apply. A game set early on in the response would focus on balancing reacting and over-reacting, and the cost of committing resources. Later in the response we would know how the response was going, and how fast and far the disease had progressed. Given the natural inclination of policy makers to wait before committing resources or disrupting society it is likely things probably are not going as well as they should. At that stage the emphasis changes at the strategic level from resource allocation to communications. How will the various responsible government departments organize an effective communications strategy about the response, and work to change the overall course of a less than perfect response?

Where you place the players in the timeline for your strategic game will affect the decisions that they are forced to make. While this is true for any game, it is at its most intense at the strategic level where issues of attribution, retaliation, communication, and blame come into play.

What are your options for mechanics in a strategic level game? Strategic games can range from large-scale National Security Decision-Making (NSDM) games to small events held around a table. The mechanics you use should take into account that most strategic level games are about senior leaders making decisions.

Strategic games for disease response tend to focus on a couple of objectives:

- *Whole of government approach.* In addition to the interagency process this approach incorporates state, local, and legislative aspects. It will also engage with media and economic impacts. NSDMs fall into this category.

- *Exhibition games.* Games on major disasters are often used to highlight issues to not only the response system, but also to the media and the public. These games are generally more streamlined than an NSDM, they involve current or former government officials, and they have a high media profile with video, social media, and other media integrated into the publicizing of the game, often even as it's occurring.

- *International games.* Gaming can be used to bring together decision-makers from different countries in order to practice and learn about a coordinated international disease response. While these games are often operationally focused, they straddle the line between operational and strategic because many of the decisions that need to be made are related to national strategy and policy. For example, should borders be closed? Should vaccine be shared? Those move beyond the operational level to the strategic.

- *Key leader games.* These games are designed to set up important issues, like pandemic response, for senior leaders, like head's of state, to discuss. The games are often very structured, with leaders coming with prepared positions and agendas to present to the assembled. Preparations start well in advance and need to be vetted with the leaders' staffs. The staffs will work through the issues that will be raised in the game and pre-brief the leader on their positions and recommended response. This avoids embarrassing situations, most of the time.

The decisions you encounter in strategic games include: [227]

- *Policy.* Should we do something like let the cruise ships, with multiple cases onboard, dock? What are the trade-offs medically, ethically, and politically?

- *Messaging.* In disease response operations senior leaders and their staffs spend a lot of time on trying to find the right message to give to the public. There are an enormous number of trade-offs, and the wrong message, as we have seen from a lot of recent operations, can backfire against the administration. Poor messaging can cost lives.

- *Operational.* Senior political leaders can have significant input into operational details. This has been the case with recent operations.

- *Budgetary and economic.* Response operations cost money and can have economic and social impact depending on the measures taken. These considerations draw in the legislative branch of government as well as the business community.

---

[227] All of these are based on examples in both real-world and game response operations.

- *Capabilities.* One challenge in response operations is often identifying all of the various capabilities that exist to respond. In some cases, agencies may wish to avoid their capabilities being used either because of cost, precedent, or an unwillingness to be exposed to the public.

- *Authorities and regulations.* A function of the senior levels of government that impacts responses are the authorities for various actions. The most common example of this is quarantine, how it can be imposed and who can impose it. But there is a vast landscape of authority issues that can cause trouble. These range from who can direct traffic to licensing and liability.

If you know what the key decisions are you can build your scenario to focus the players on them. For example, if issues of legal policy, quarantine, and international law are things that you want to explore in your game, then including a cruise ship component would potentially exercise all of those elements. Making the disease plague, which is reportable in a maritime environment, would give the players additional challenges.

If those issues are not the focus of the game, then you can just as easily leave the cruise ships out as they will become a potential distraction for the players. Real world events encompass the entire range of policy, economic, and capacities questions, but if you observe a real-world response only some of those issues become highlighted for policy-makers. No one said much about cruise ships during the SARS outbreak, but during the recent COVID outbreak they were a major component of the early response phase. Likewise, the cross-border coordination on SARS was important between the US and Canada, while COVID did not focus on that issue.

Picking the type of game involves:

- How many players must you have, or how many can you recruit? The more players you have the more effective it will be to divide them into teams and smaller groups. This tends to push you toward a seminar game, while fewer players push you toward a tabletop.[228]

- What are the decisions the players will be making? Are the decisions focused on one, unique, group of people such as the National Security Council? Or does there need to be collaboration between different groups?

- What is the relative seniority of the players? In a game where one individual vastly "outranks" all of the others then the expectation will be that the high-ranking individual will have an important role. The converse works as well—can you get individuals senior enough to be familiar with the kind of decisions you need?

- How structured is the problem? By "structured" I mean how specific is the set of objective questions the game is trying to ask. In a highly structured game, there will be a set of topics or decisions that simply must be made. With fewer topics, or a desire to understand what topics are important, the decisions will be more up to the players. The more specific the topics and detailed the processes involved the more structured the game and the greater the influence of the game Controller. This is to make sure the game stays on track and the specific subjects get addressed.

The materials you provide the players should also reflect the role in government that they are playing. Senior leaders don't get a lot of detail, rather the information is synthesized by staffs and the key points brought forward. Guess what? In games like this the game designer (or someone they designate as victim) are the staff. So, it is up to you to make sure the players get the information synthesized for the right level (including missing or incomplete information).

The pace of the game should not allow for extended discussions that almost all senior players, especially retired mid-level government officials, like to engage in. Ending a discussion early is better than letting it range over topics irrelevant to the game. This can be difficult: a good facilitator will be able to maintain focus on the topic and cut off spurious discussions in a tabletop format. In a larger seminar or NSDM format control will need to monitor the game and identify potentially disruptive, or simply long winded, players.

There are a couple of ways to deal with disruptive players:

---

[228] But, you say, shouldn't game objectives determine the number of players? Remember from earlier: game objectives are just one of two determinants in game design. The other is constraints. Often you are constrained in one fashion or another to a given number of players. Your design has to be able to adapt to constraints.

- *Give them a specific task.* This works well when the person has a particular set of skills or interest, that can then be brought back into the game in some sort of controlled fashion.

- *Bring them into control.* They can be a special senior advisor or help construct something harmless. This plays to the player's ego (which is often the issue) and lets them contribute to the overall play of the game.

- *Take them aside and explain the situation.* This may or may not work and should be resorted to when you can't find a way to integrate them into the game naturally.

- *Ask them to leave.* This can be tricky and should only be used in cases where someone is being deliberately and extensively disruptive. However, there is more than one way to leave the game. They could go off into the "special" debating cell where they can speak with all their peers endlessly on topics irrelevant to the game. They can also become observers, providing their wisdom and insights directly into the game report.

I have emphasized the seniority of the players in strategic games because that is often the most challenging aspect of this type of game. Unfortunately, it is even more challenging to have players who don't know how policy decisions are made at the highest levels of government. So, you trade off the danger of seniority for the liabilities of ignorance.

Operational Games

Operational level games are the most common type of professional game used by government. Strategic games are almost equally common, but many of them are sponsored by quasi-government agencies and educational institutions working for government, as opposed to directly created by government personnel or contractors. Operational games are found throughout the examples in this book because the questions that they raise are often the most interesting ones for those who respond to events:

- How will different agencies work together? What are other organizations going to do different from what we have planned for them to do?

- What resources will we need during an operation and how do those resources compare to what we've got?

- What has not been considered in our existing plans and preparations?

- Can we design a different organization, process, or plan so that we are more efficient, successful, or collaborative?

- Maybe we could show that the other organizations in this department will not cooperate during an emergency, and leadership will do something about it! (Yes, you can; no, they won't.)

We can divide operational games according to the game questions:

- Organizational. Who is in charge?

- Planning. What is our plan?

- Execution. Can we make our plan work in the real world?

Operational level games exist in the gray zone between extremely detailed tactical games and the more abstract policy or strategic games. To drive the needed organizational interactions, they require you feed them detail in the scenario, injects, and adjudication. Players need that detail in order to lose themselves in the game, to create the impression that the game is "real." This is a necessity in operational level games because all of the organizational shenanigans that happen in the real world won't happen unless the game seems "real" to the players. If it's real then the players are more likely to exhibit their real-world behaviors, biases, and objectives.

This is great, except you are playing with people whose job it is to know the operational detail.

This is the biggest challenge you face as a designer in operational level games. Your players know their operational details, because it's their job to know them. They understand the plans, and more importantly how the plans are supposed to work. The game has to at least represent the facts of their plan, and acknowledge any assumptions, or you are essentially criticizing your players ability to do their jobs. This is a very tricky enterprise to say the least.

The best way designers rise to the challenge of operational level games is by creating the environment where the players can compete over plans, authorities, and resources. Players tend to believe other players, particularly when they are professionals in the field, more than they believe the game designer. It is also beneficial that they are not always focused on the game designer or controller.

So how do you build the kind of operational detail you need into games? You can:

- *Do research.* Open-source intelligence gathering (OSINT) is a skill that will serve you well as a game designer. Most organizations have information available online, and the subject-matter area or disease will usually have an extensive literature. Giving yourself a background in General Accounting Office (GAO) reports, Congressional testimony, and think-tank pieces on the subject are the first place to start your research.

- *Talk to experts.* In most cases you will be doing the game for an organization that works in the field and is the subject of the game. Let's take a game on hospital capacity. It will likely be done for an organization that knows stuff about hospitals. Use the expertise of people within that organization. It is important when doing this that you be very specific. "So how, exactly, do capacity decisions get made, when are they made, who makes them, what data do they use, who do they tell about the decision, etc." These specific questions will drill down into the detail that you need for the game. They will also give you an idea for what the next question should be, for example, "it seems like there is a substantial emphasis on profit, how does that factor in?" If the questions become more awkward, and the answers more revealing, then you are doing it right.

- *Talk to the players ahead of time.* There is often the idea that revealing the scenario or game idea to the players before the game will somehow cause them to 'cheat.' Experience indicates this is not true. Players are busy, they don't listen, often forget, and in the game, they get swept up in the job and forget what you told them. Or all of the above. Asking the players how they will act in certain situations can be quire revealing. "Oh, we never use the Hospital Associations plan, that was just made up to make the state happy. Instead, we are going to do incident management off of the regional hospital's plan, that usually works much better." If you don't want to talk to the players, talk to people who have similar jobs as they do within the organization.

- *Use subject-matter experts (SMEs).* If neither the players nor the sponsor knows anything about the question, you can refer to various types of experts to support you. The easiest are those referred by the sponsor and players, they will have a better understanding of local detail. Adjacent organizations often have the kind of detail you are looking for. In the case of the hospital problem, it might be a pharmaceutical association or the director of local emergency management. You can also go to academics, or other professionals in the field, but these will be unlikely to have the kind of local experience that you really need.

The most important thing is that you actually listen to the experts. You need to not only understand what they are telling you, but what they are telling you between the lines, and what they are not telling you. Research will help you predict these omissions, as will experience. But nothing really beats carefully listening for those things that will make your game interesting, and important, to the players and sponsor. These can usually be identified because they involve:

- Conflict, especially rivalries or competing ambitions.

- Deviation from norms and standards.

- Resources, especially funding.

- Anything else that creates tensions within or between organizations.

In operational games we often focus a lot on the action, the operators and responders. For most medical games that is the medical and administrative staffs at hospitals and the public-health professionals. But there are other elements that matter at the operational level and often do not get considered. These include:

- *Mental health.* SAMHSA is a major component of HHS and crisis-response mental-health care is an element of almost all response operations.

- *Legal.* Legal issues with health-care responses in the United States can be tricky, complicated, and often limiting. For example, New York State had to modify medical licenses in order for out of state doctors to practice there during the COVID-19 response.[229]

- *Indian Health Services (IHS).* IHS is a component of DHS and provides tribal health services and public health response on tribal lands.[230] If an event spills onto tribal land then the IHS will have some responsibility and requirements to provide public health and health care. It will also mean that the legal issues will multiply.

- *Other functions.* The Public Health Service also provides health care in some federal situations such as social services for detained migrant children. They also staff the Immigration and Customs Enforcement (ICE) Health Services Corps (HSC) which provides health care to detained migrant adults.[231]

Understanding these other functions of HHS and PHS can help you construct accurate and believable public-health scenarios. If you include migration, or emergencies associated with tribal areas, you will definitely need to account for them. This is what I mean by operational games requiring an attention to detail, not in terms of the disease but in the overall organizational response as well.

In our operational melioidosis game we can begin to anticipate how the various components will react before we actually play the game. As patients come into the system, we can anticipate that it will go through a series of phases, from recognition "we have a problem" to initial response "put them in that empty ward" to long-term relief "let's set up a system to effectively deliver IV antibiotics every 12 hours to all these patients" to recovery "this disease has a long tail, how will we deal with this as a chronic disease over the next 20 years?"

This allows us to adjust my disease parameters to better match what we want to do in the game. If we want to push the diagnostic portion of the game, we will have a detailed breakdown of how the disease will present. That will vary and not always involve emergency rooms. Some urgent care facilities may not be hooked up to the health surveillance system, or if commuters go home to a different public-health region, then coordination on the initial recognition of the event will become complex. On the other hand, if we really want to push the response phase, we can increase the overall exposure rates, and the exposure dosing. This will give me a lot of initial patients and slam the hospital and care system before they are really able to collect personnel and supplies for an effective response.

Understanding how the systems works, where the key vulnerabilities are, and how the disease parameters will play into those vulnerabilities makes the difference between a good game and a great game. If we can pitch the game at the point where their plans matter, but are not sufficient, to solve the problem players will be more engaged, and have to really evaluate whether their plans work. It makes the difference between a game where the plan is simply exercised and one where the players are integral component to solving the problem. In the latter case the players have to react to something they did not expect, then adapt and think on their feet.

Tactical games

Tactical games are the public health games that most resemble military wargames. Here we are focused on the mechanical details of executing an operation. Tactical games can be defined by:

- *Scale.* If the game is confined to one element of an overall response it can be considered tactical. A game on a vaccination line would be an example of a tactical game defined by scale.

- *Level of decisions.* One organization's operational level game may be another's tactical game. What a county government will do during an event can be considered tactical from the perspective of the State or Federal government. Tactical games defined on level tend to focus on the end rung of an organization and how it will respond. For example, you could have a tactical level game on an FBI investigation focused on the actions of the field office. While the FBI is a federal agency it has tactical roles executed by its various subordinate elements.

---

[229] http://www.op.nysed.gov/COVID-19_EO.html - and that is not the only case where medical licensing has been an issue in disaster response operations.

[230] www.ihs.gov

[231] You can use this in a game by having an outbreak start in a detention facility, which will immediately introduce a seam between federal and state response processes.

- *Time.* Tactical games can look at very small units of time. For example, what is the response during the first hours of an outbreak, as the hospitals and systems, even at the operational level, begin to realize what is happening and prepare their actions.

Thus, we can have a both county health response, as seen in Chapter 12, and a vaccination line be considered tactical games.

In building tactical games the designer is confronted by a need to not only know the plans and processes involved, but also the practical considerations of the response. This can mean developing analytical models to describe physical or process events or measuring out distances and travel times to understand when various events will occur. You use this understanding to structure the time, space, and rules for the game.

For example, in the case of the vaccination line the designer would be well advised to do some basic math on the queuing problems involved so that they will have some idea of how many people will be where during the game. If the parking lot can hold 100 cars, and each car on average carries 1.5 individuals, then you can expect a full parking lot to mean that 150 people will be somewhere in the various queues in the vaccination line. Assuming a flow rate of 15 people per 15 minutes through the process that means 60 people per hour can arrive at the parking lot without causing backups of traffic or annoyed "customers." Of course, if the word has gotten out, and its life or death, a lot more than 60 may arrive per hour, and you have not yet considered foot or bus traffic. Doing some basic math and estimates prior to the event will save you a lot of grief.

In addition, doing the analysis on tactical games up front also provides you with smart questions to ask the experienced public health and safety professionals you will be working with. If you come in clueless as to the parking problem, then you will not garner much respect, or help, from the people who have volunteered (almost always it's a volunteer) to give you information in support of your game. However, if you have at least half thought through the basics, they will assume you know a lot more about the subject than you probably do, and be more willing to help you understand the details of their particular system. Which is what you really need.

Research on tactical games is indispensable not just for the game itself, but also to support pre-game design conversations with subject matter experts.

Unlike many, but not all, operational and strategic public health games, tactical games have issues of position, movement, and location. This means you will need a map, and often pieces to represent various elements in the game. In the case of a game on a vaccination clinic you might have a large map of the facility with pieces representing different kind of patients, medical professionals, data entry and support professionals, and security. You could even personalize the patients (and others) with cards describing them in detail.

For example, you have a family enter the clinic. There is a card associated with the family that describes one adult female, who only speaks Tagalog (Pilipino), who is diabetic, along with three children of various ages two of whom have evidence of possible abuse. The children speak English. This will give the players a variety of challenges, involving both moving them through the vaccination process, but also through the social services and translation requirements.

Tactical games also often need to manage time in a structured way so that players, and control, know what is happening when. This can involve structured turns or moves, where each move represents a fixed amount of time an all of the elements of a game update during the turn. In the case of the vaccination clinic your queuing models provide the basic number of people at each station as a function of time and player decisions. You run a discreet version of the model to update the situation within the clinic according to what the players decide to do, how long it would take to implement, and how it would impact other elements of the operation.

So, for example, players implement a new step where some vaccination patients are separated out for additional screening based on illness or other factors. They may see mental health or social service professionals as well. This will add time to their residency in the line, while decreasing load on other parts of the line. No matter what the parking lot will get backed up.

In tactical games the scenarios will likely need to be detailed in ways similar to what we just described. You may need to know the backstory of every patient, even though most of them will not present a challenge to the players. The ones that do present a challenge may have been derived from your discussions with the people assigned to help you prior to the game. As with operational game players, they live the response and events every day, and have likely encountered any number of unique or challenging cases in their experience. They can be directly lifted into the game or provide an inspiration for scenario elements.

Often in our experience the game designer will know enough about a problem to provide a basic scenario, but the "ah-ha" elements of a scenario come from the actual practitioners. And no matter how you get to the unique elements, realizing that something might happen often inspires an entire line of thought in the game as you think through the various ramifications and requirements associated with a problem. For example, in the case above, what, exactly, might the clinicians do with an indicator of abuse? In many states medical professionals have to report such a suspicion, but a mass vaccination line is significantly different than a clinical setting. How would they go about it? More importantly, what other things might they encounter that would require some sort of reporting or counseling that have nothing to do with what is happening at the vaccination line, but requires them ethically or legally to take action?

Once you ask one question (abuse) many other questions can occur as you begin to think the scenario problem through.

Most professional tactical games do not have rigid rules the way many hobby boardgames do. This is because there is typically a professional facilitator working with the players so that the players are not burdened with understanding a series of complicated rules for a game, they may play only one time. In addition, the facilitators make sure that the game is played "correctly" as a mis-understanding of some critical rule can seriously affect game outcomes.

However, just because the players don't have rules to abide by that does not mean the facilitator/controllers don't have rules they use. In professional games this is termed "adjudication" and as it implies control "adjudicates" the player actions.

The analysis you did up front in the game, in order to understand the basic dynamics and mathematics of what is going on, will help with adjudication during the game. In the case of the vaccination line game a basic spreadsheet models of queues will allow you to add a queue when players introduce social services or mental health into the flow. This allows for adjudication of the effects on the rest of the game elements.

In a tactical game, even one of something as seemingly simple as a vaccination clinic, can require the controllers to adjudicate things they never expected to. For example, what if a security guard has to tackle someone? What happens?

There are several ways to deal with these unexpected "ad-hoc" adjudications:

- Estimation. Based on what you know, or assume, what is a logical set of outcomes for the situation? In the case of the security guard the tackle is either successful, or not, depending on what the geometry and physics of the situation are. If the guard is after a quick track star and starts from 100 feet away on a stage sitting down, it will likely fail. If the guard is standing next to the individual, who is already mobility impaired, then they will just grab hold of them.

- Random. You can always roll a die and see what the roll tells you. On a six sided die a "one" could represent success and a "six" failure. So, if you roll a "3" the guard might successfully catch the individual, but knocks something valuable over in the process. A "six" might mean that they also catch the individual, but both are not seriously injured and require medical treatment.

- Other rule sets. There are many games that describe what they would term "grappling combat" and give values you could use to determine the outcome.[232]

- Inductive or necessity. In some cases, you simply want to have something happen in the game. Perhaps you want to introduce trauma injuries and police actions into the vaccination clinic, so you rule that the tackle produces them. If, on the other hand, this is a distraction, you can easily rule that things get sorted out quickly and peaceably and everyone returns to their normal business.

- Consensus. This can range from having all the players discuss an adjudication to one or more subject matter experts (SME) deciding what the outcome would be. There are advantages to having the players discuss an important outcome but adding any sort of committee action to an already complicated and involved game can significantly lengthen the game.

---

[232] For our grappling example see Tactical Studies Rules (TSR). (1990) *Boot Hill 3rd edition*. Typically these rules are too complicated to use in fast-paced professional games where it can be difficult to stop, page through a bunch of rules, figure out modifiers and to-hit numbers, and then roll for the outcome.

Tactical games almost always require the designer to have a good understanding of the details of the problem. This happens through analysis and the input of those who have done the task before. These inputs allow for a detailed and specific scenario to be developed that provides the kind of granularity necessary in these sorts of games. It also assists in adjudication, as specific player actions will require results assigned to them based on physics and the reality of the situation.

Chapter 14: Mental Health

The time is: 0830 31 July.

The Assistant Secretary for Mental Health and Substance Abuse looked around their office at everyone in the meeting. The situation was not only getting out of hand, it had made all the cable news networks. The Secretary would probably be calling shortly to prepare for a trip to the White House. Already Congressional staff were beginning to ask questions. The monthly tracking report on virtually every measure of mental health was suddenly heading in a dramatically wrong direction. Indicators of substance abuse, depression, domestic violence, and calls for crisis counseling had doubled in the last month. The ongoing pandemic had isolated the already lonely, and increased unemployment and hardship. The current patchwork of grants, research tools, and efforts would not be enough. They needed to integrate across the organization. How, exactly, they would pull together tribal, mental health, substance prevention, and other efforts from across the organization was anyone's guess. But they better have an idea before the Secretary called.

Objective

This game explores the inner workings of the Substance Abuse and Mental Health Services Administration as they reorganize in response to a pandemic. The premise of the game is fictional, built to represent a possible set of objectives and goals for a game dealing with SAMHSA.[233] The goal is to increase overall delivery of mental health and substance-abuse services in a way that is coordinated between private providers, grant recipients (clinics, many serving tribal communities), state and local agencies, and SAMSHA. While coordination currently occurs, the goal is to build a mental health delivery system that is able to manage and track mental health patients across different social and health services, in order to treat both the symptoms (substance abuse, for example) as we all the underlying causes (isolation, homelessness, job loss, etc.). This will require several actions that may not be terribly popular, including changing the way grants are issued, how insurance covers mental health and substance abuse treatment, and how mental health professionals integrate into housing and food assistance programs. This will require both legislative as well as organizational changes. The goal is to identify both types of changes, and then advance a comprehensive plan through the administration.[234] The advantage of the game is policy makers can ask any question and experiment in the blame free environment of a game.

Background

Pandemics can cause disruption in social systems, particularly if movement control or isolation is imposed on large segments of the population.[235] The challenge is made worse by the inability of providers to see patients face-to-face, instead substituting telemedicine.[236] The isolation caused by movement controls, the effects of a depressed economy, and the general worries surrounding the pandemic can increase the overall rate of substance abuse or mental health issues. In this scenario we posit that during the middle of a pandemic, one that has resulted in extended and repeated impositions of movement controls, that mental health and substance abuse issues have spiked to levels that they have become a matter for national interest. The question is: what are Health and Human Services (HHS) and SAMSHA going to do about it?

---

[233] We are making up a scenario and set of goals and objectives to illustrate how a game like this may be constructed. This is a fictional game, and a fictional scenario.

[234] This objective has no basis in the reality of how services are currently provided. It represents a plausible objective that you would see for a game involving a government agency. We do not mean to imply any deficiencies in SAMSHA or indeed any interest or ability in SAMSHA's part to engage in efforts along these lines. It is entirely possible that some of the gaps we posit here have already been identified and addressed by SAMSHA. Or they may not exist in the first place.

[235] While this was not obvious prior to the outbreak of COVID-19, it is obvious now. Centers for Medicare and Medicaid Services (CMS) and Substance Abuse and Mental Health Services Administration (SAMHSA). (29 Jun 2020) *Leveraging Existing Health and Disease Management Programs to Provide Mental Health Services and Substance Use Disorder Resources during the COVID-19 Public Health Emergency (PHE).*

[236] SAMHSA. (7 May 2020) *Considerations for the Care and Treatment of Mental and Substance Use Disorders in the COVID-19 Epidemic.*

We posit that a whole of government approach is desired, along with partnerships with public providers and insurance companies. This partnership will go beyond mental health to attempt to provide a 360-degree view of the problem. The challenge is that there are multiple stakeholders involved, from individual providers to insurance companies, and that these organizations all have their own agendas. The game is designed to bring together these disparate stakeholders and attempt to find solutions that everyone can endorse, support, and live with. Of course, the solutions also need to actually address the problem.

Products from the game could include:

- A reorganization of the SAMSHA grant program to focus grants on enablers for this 360-degree approach toward mental health.

- Identifying how an expansion of the SAMSHA budget to include both grant and services administration programs would increase value.

- New concepts for research in support of the 360-degree approach to mental health

- Building a program within HHS to link departmental and interagency responses to the problem. Specifically, the goal is to link with programs in the Department of Education, Housing and Urban Development, and the Social Security Administration. Links also need to be established or enhances with programs inside HHS such the Centers for Medicare and Medicaid Services.

- A public messaging program integrated with an HHS "one voice" concept as well as CDC and White House messaging.

- A plan to engage with the Congress on legislation for items that HHS cannot change directly.

This is a relatively straightforward role-playing game set against a current, and ongoing, scenario. That means that you would not have to provide the players a lot of detail on the pandemic, only the guidance and direction from the Secretary regarding how to re-imagine mental health programs. You would also need to provide data on the immediate mental health situation, especially the media, information, and political environment.

Players

We are going to limit the number of players. The more players you have in a game the more viewpoints will be present and the results will possibly be richer in content. However, the more players you have, the longer the game takes, and you will be able to address fewer issues in detail. We have also discussed large-scale role-playing games in several of the examples, here we want to illustrate a smaller, tabletop, game.

For this game to have the greatest impact we will need players from the actual agencies and organizations mentioned. If players have to engage in role-playing it requires a lot more background material for the "naive" players. This includes information about what the organizations do and what are their interests and equities. We want to avoid this problem by bringing in players from the actual agencies involved. We also want to bring in outside participants from various mental health providers and grant recipients.

An around-the-table game's set of players would include:

- SAMSHA (one player each)
    - Office of the Assistant Secretary
    - Office of Communications
    - Center for Substance Abuse and prevention
    - Center for Mental Health Services
- CMS – one player
- Indian Health Services – one player
- Grant recipients – one player with grant experience
- Mental health professional – one player representing mental health services providers
- Insurance industry – one or two players representing the insurance industry

- Senior leadership review panel – these are not players, rather this group meets to hear what the initial outcome of the work is

That is a total of nine players plus the review panel. It is likely that others, for example the office in charge of grant programs, may be needed. A total of twelve players is not unlikely once the game is vetted through the organization.

Game concept

A common problem in around-the-table games is developing a problem sufficiently compelling so as to get the players working on the topic, but not so overwhelming as to be out of the scope of action of a small number of participants. One game design technique that is often used is to have the players play as a part of some sort of ad-hoc task force working on the problem.

In this case we will assign the government players the role of a task force that is working on an overhaul of how services are provided during a pandemic. Their task is to present a spectrum of options across all of the different mental health and substance abuse services and organizations. The other players—the other organizations represented in the game—have a similar charter but only for their particular organization. They can collaborate with SAMSHA and become part of SAMSHA's task force (assuming organizational restrictions will permit it) or not as they choose. This allows some agency for the other players and allows different points of view to be developed.

The game will progress through the following stages:

- All players will meet to understand the rules and flow of the game. The venue would likely be a large conference room plus one or two smaller ones for breakout sessions.

- Players are given the scenario and their tasking, to come up with a preliminary plan. Game materials include:
  o An introduction to the game (game book).
  o A briefing on the current state of the pandemic (it should be severe enough to have triggered several shutdowns and widespread unemployment).
  o A briefing on the latest mental health and substance abuse statistics.
  o Newsfeed (either print or video) making it clear that the media has picked up on the mental health aspects and something must be done by the administration.

- The players will then self-organize, with the SAMSHA players falling under the Office of the Assistant Secretary.

- Players plan, and possibly interact in different ways depending on what is being discussed. For example, supposed that changes are required to the way mental health professionals are regulated so that insurance companies can expand insurance coverage for mental health issues. Then all parties will need to have a discussion about the effects of those changes.

- Players present their plan to the senior leadership review panel – along with the other players – and receive feedback and reaction

- Players modify the plan according to what happened in the review panel.

This is a very different game from a response game because it focuses on planning as opposed to action. This is not unusual for organizational games where the scenario is designed to drive a planning process and the ultimate product is the plan as opposed to insights or a set of player actions. These games can be significantly less dramatic, but they allow for all stakeholders in a situation to participate since they are "off the books" and not really an official planning action.

By bringing in the senior leaders we focus the players' actions and give them some meaning beyond just briefing each other on a plan at the end of the day. We would like the senior leaders to be representatives from both the White House, Office of Management and Budget, and Congress: think deputy White House policy director, senior Congressional aid, and a mid-level manager at OMB. But they could also be senior leaders from within HHS, SAMSHA, or CMS if SAMSHA does not want to expose the exercise to the White House or the Hill[237].

The plan will likely be in briefing format, so the venue will need to support computers, printers, and broadband.

The reason we did not do this as a directed discussion or matrix game (which we will talk about later) is because it is about planning, not taking actions. So, games where you ask people what they would do in a situation do not make sense for this kind of game. Instead giving people a problem, space to discuss it, coordinate about it, and test it against something (in this case senior leaders) is a better concept.

This game would work for a 1 day or shorter game. The time would depend on how fast you thought the players could build the concept, and whether you had people from the White House and Hill to vet the plan. Higher echelon people mean you need to design a shorter game.

You could replace the senior leaders with an execution phase, where you had to get your plan through Congress and the White House, then implement it amongst the various HHS, CMS, SAMSHA, grantee, and civilian groups. This would work better as a two-day game, even if both days are only half days. In this case players would take one day to come up with a plan, and then attempt to implement it in a larger game the second day, with players representing all the affected stake holders. This would allow for more realistic jockeying, complaining, and stonewalling as the second day players would not have been briefed on the plan. This would give the sponsor some idea of the challenges they might face in implementing the plan.

And that is the ultimate goal of this game: to give those responsible for implementing the new policy and operational concepts a chance to "test fly" them before they actually build them. In any organizational environment, but particularly a governmental or interagency environment, there will be all sorts of unknown challenges and issues that come up. Being able to deal with them in a relatively benign environment where the outcomes don't really count can provide a lot of help to those responsible for putting together a plan.

Execution

As we discussed in the previous session this will be an "around the table" game similar to what we did for the melioidosis game in chapter 12. In this instance the game will proceed according to events that happen instead of a timeline. First players will need to come up with the task force's proposed plan. This will rely heavily on the existing laydown for the scenario, control will be able to clarify the situation but won't have a lot of leeway to introduce new events or challenges into the game after it starts.

Turn 1

The first turn will consist of the players self-organizing into task groups in order to address the challenges presented by the ongoing pandemic. Players will need to identify how mental health research should change, and how the granting and funding process will need to change with it. They may also propose better integration of mental health into other aspects of the response, and perhaps a reorganization. Players should eventually reconvene as one panel and discuss all of the various proposals that have been developed. Control can facilitate this discussion, but often one or more players take the lead. These can be representatives of the game sponsor, or simply players with strong leadership drives.

Once all of the players have discussed and debated the plan, they will need to turn the plan into a presentation. There are a couple of ways to do this, none of which are very satisfactory. You can assign one or two players the job of doing the presentation, or you can have a scribe and everyone talk about what should be in the presentation. When doing this control should be aware of equality issues and ensure that the role of scribe or slide developer does not automatically fall on the youngest, or female, players.

Turn 2

Players will then present the results of their planning to a higher-ranking panel where the plan will be discussed. This is where control facilitates the conversation if they can. Sometimes senior panels can be difficult to control, and other times the sponsor wants to have control when their seniors are in the room. But if control is called on to facilitate then the most important job for control is to keep the overall objective in focus. The goal is to get senior feedback on whether plans are implementable, and, if not, what needs to change. A good facilitator will

---

[237] US Senate.

be on the lookout for subtle indicators that the plan has strayed across political 'red lines', and the facilitator will work to better define what those 'red lines' are and how the plan can adapt to them[238].

Often with panels the panelists will attempt to filibuster. That is fine, as long as the panel ultimately makes the necessary decisions, or refers those decisions back to the players for more or better planning. Hopefully some of the ideas the players had will be seen as implementable by the panel, while others will require re-work.

Turn 3

At this point in the game there are two possibilities; the panel has given comprehensive and interesting advice to the players and they are charged with updating, expanding, and building implementations for what they presented. Or the panel has taken further work off the table by either accepting all of the players recommendations, or, worse, rejecting them without much hope of any sort of way forward. Control needs to be prepared for both possibilities.

In the first case, control will simply help the lead players structure the rest of their time and identify changes that need to be made to the plan. Once key issues have been identified the players go off and refine the plan based on the panel input, build the final plan, and present it to each other for critique. This will then flow into the hotwashup. Again, the role of control is to keep the players on track, both in terms of what they are working and in terms of time.

The second case is much harder for control to deal with. This is a "pencils down" situation for the players and can end the game. If the panel has been supportive and said everything is perfect, now is the time for the players to begin to build the implementation plan. Control can facilitate a group discussion on how the plan will work in the real world. This will likely identify areas that need further work, or issues that have not yet been raised. It is likely that a "great" plan will have upset at least a few of the players and their organizations, and this turn is just the time to try and deal with those upsets. Because control participated in the design of the game they will know where the difficult spots are, and can bring them out in facilitation.

If the worst has occurred, and the senior panel has been discouraging or unhelpful, then the Controller and sponsor need to act to have the players revise their plan into some other alternative that may either be more acceptable, or more compelling. It is at this point that control may quit their controller role and become more of a mentor and analyst. After all, because control is part of the design team, they understand the problem in detail and should be able to help the players think through another course of action. Likewise, the sponsor, hoping to get a way forward out of the game should be motivated to roll up their sleeves and participate.

The "pencils down" case is rare, most people want a game to succeed and want to have a good outcome. However, if there is a mis-match between sponsor expectations and the organizational reality, or if the panel is simply unaware of the reason for their tasking, then these sorts of situations can arise. Control should be prepared for them and work to mitigate them whenever possible. Potential mitigation techniques could be having a chat with important panel members prior to the game. During the design phase these chats would serve to introduce the panel to the game while at the same time surfacing any issues before they became problems the day of the game. You cannot rely on your sponsor to always know what the challenges are. They may be overly optimistic, or simply unable to confront senior leaders in the way an outside game designer can.

---

[238] Political red lines are political stances that cannot be changed due to the democratically leaders reflecting the views of their electorate.

Chapter 15: Plans and Processes for Disease Response

Here we continue to alternate between chapters that discuss game design, exercises, and chapters that discuss public health response through the lens of gaming. In this chapter we focus on the planning and processes that go into any disease response.

Any game on response operations will likely focus on the response plan that everyone is supposed to use. The US Federal Government, and almost all state and local governments, have plans for how to respond to various kinds of events. These plans, for the most part, are conceptual, assigning roles and responsibilities, not detailing every action that needs to be done, but giving the overall framework for the operation. Because these plans are gamed and exercised almost continuously[239] the players of a game dealing with disease response will expect that the plans and their processes will be reflected in the game design.

Plans are usually seen as adaptable, being guidelines that flex to the needs of the particular response operation. Deviate too far from the plan and everyone can become confused. Stick to the plan rigidly and you can fail with the response. The challenge is between standardization and creativity, between assessment and innovation, and between testing and creating. The exercises and games put on by DHS and other government agencies tend toward the test/assess/standardize end of the spectrum because those types of games can at least be seen to be quantitively assessed and compared, thus providing "product" for the funds and effort expended. This has gone a long way in standardizing the response processes and making sure everyone knows what to expect and do in an operation.

Games can also challenge teams to deal with unexpected or unanticipated events. They can ask the players to figure out how to flex, but not break the plan. This involves more than assessing whether a particular plan or system is in place, followed, and properly resourced. Games can challenge the very nature of the plan and extend or explore the players' ability to adapt to unforeseen circumstances. However, if you want to do a game that expands the players' world, you first have to understand a little bit about that world. And it is usually a world dominated by plans, authorities, responsibilities, and capabilities. And bureaucracies, lots of bureaucracies.

These plans determine who talks to whom, and who is responsible for what. They are how organizations work.

Disease Response Operations

The most basic distinction is between response operations and other types of routine operations. In response operations someone is responding to something: a disaster, emergency, humanitarian crisis, famine, mass migration, technical disaster, or disease outbreak. Disaster-response operations typically go through phases: response, relief, recovery, and mitigation. In this section we attempt to map these phases onto disease response, with imperfect results. [240] The reason we do this is to enable us to discuss disease response in the context of all of the other response plans in government. Disease response doesn't quite fit into this model due to its extended timelines for monitoring and surveillance prior or in the early phases of a disease outbreak. If we identify a disease outbreak early and act, we can prevent it, which is hard to do with many other types of natural disasters.

The response phase comes first in a disaster. The response phase comes right after the event occurs. The focus in the response phase is on stopping the immediate threat to life and health. In the aftermath of a hurricane this would be looking for survivors and treating the injured. In a disease response this can be an extended period of time, depending on the nature of the disease, when it is identified, when actions begin occurring, and how many are affected. [241]

After the response phase comes the relief phase, during which responding organizations attempt to stabilize the situation and restore some normalcy. For a hurricane, the relief phase would involve setting up tents and providing clean water and supplies. For disease-response operations this would merge with the response phase,

---

[239] For example, FEMA/DHS has the National Exercise Program (https://www.fema.gov/national-exercise-program) along with providing grants and funds to states and communities to hold their own exercises and games. They even provide guidelines for conducting exercises (https://www.fema.gov/hseep).

[240] For one of the best discussions of the disaster process see Kent, Randolph. (1987) *The Anatomy of Disaster Relief.* For health planning see: Rose, Dale A et al. (2017) "The Evolution of Public Health Emergency Management as a Field of Practice." *American journal of public health* vol. 107,S2 S126-S133. doi:10.2105/AJPH.2017.303947

[241] Even for something like pneumonic plague there is a low baseline level of incidents that will occur during a year.

when hospital capacity is being extended and threats to other aspects of national infrastructure from the disease are being managed.

The relief phase is followed by recovery, where everyone attempts to restore the environment to the same condition it was in before the event. The recovery phase involves rebuilding housing stocks and restoring electrical power. Finally, there is the mitigation phase, in which you prepare for the next disaster.

For disease response mitigation is a major element of the overall response. It combines surveillance with prevention and preparation. It can also merge into response as small outbreaks are identified, treated, and suppressed without the event become a larger challenge. Disease response can be seen as having a large mitigation phase, followed by an extended response, that eventually, if the disease outbreak becomes significant enough, moves into response and recovery as the medical and health systems adapt to the outbreak and begin increasing capacity and changing the way they operate.

The response phase for disease can be much longer than for a sudden onset disaster like a hurricane, and the relief phase can combine with the response phase, while the recovery phase merges with mitigation.

The phases of a disaster response play an important role in planning, resourcing, and phasing response operations. It is noteworthy that in researching this book we did not find a clear example of a full pandemic response broken into phases. As we will describe later, the World Health Organization (WHO) Pandemic Phases focus heavily on the detection and prevention work, with little definition of the response to recovery phases. As the scale of a pandemic grows the overall medical response increases, whole of government becomes involved, and it begins to look more like the response to a slow-onset disaster than it does during the early phases.

Organizations

The first building block in a response operation are the organizations that will respond. There are different ways to categorize these organizations. First is the level of US government they belong to:

- Federal

- State

- Local

- Non-governmental Organizations (NGO)/Private Volunteer Organization (PVO)

- International Governmental Organizations (IGO) (United Nations, World Health Organization, etc.)

- Private Sector Organizations (businesses)

Each of these levels will have roles, responsibilities, and plans in a response operation. They will all have different roles to play. For example, businesses can have multiple roles—some have to decide how they are going to control transmission in their workplaces while others like hospital systems or insurance companies need to contain the financial impact of the event. Businesses can also supply cleaning and protective supplies, and may be affected secondarily by closures, contamination, or public response (such as people buying lots of plastic and duct tape in case the terrorists come back). Some business-like pharmacies, medical systems, and doctors may become involved in the actual response.

In designing a game, you need to consider the role that each of these organizations play, along with the role that the public, and various sub-populations of the public (infectious, exposed, etc.) play in the game.

Plans

The US has a hierarchy of plans designed to define governmental roles during an emergency response. In this section we describe the planning framework within the United States. Not surprisingly this framework has been adopted in one form or another by many other countries, however the agencies and organizations responsible for executing a disaster response will vary widely by country.

At the topmost level we have the National Response Framework (NRF), which encompasses any potential event-response operation. Once you get below the NRF the plans we care about divide into three general types of response: disaster, disease, and bio-terrorism.

A partial list of plans includes:

- *National Response Framework.* This is a scalable plan that is designed to outline the whole-of-government approach toward any disaster. It is the framework within which other organizations can develop their plans.

- *Incident Management System (IMS).* Based on a US Fire Service operational plan, the Incident Management System is the standard way tactical units will approach an event. Even if an IMS is not fully implemented, its structure and processes inform many other plans including health planning.[242] FEMA has a National IMS (NIMS)[243] which lays down the fundamental components of an IMS: "command and coordination of incidents, resource management, and communications management." IMS also focuses on:

  o Standardization: so that different agencies and groups that show up to the same event will have a common framework for response.

  o Flexibility. The IMS is designed to be flexible enough to adapt to any situation.

  o Unity of effort. There is one commander at the incident scene, and those who show up know their roles within the framework.

- *World Health Organization Pandemic Influenza Plan.*[244] As noted above this plan focuses more on monitoring, surveillance, and threat-escalation decision points than on the details of the national and international response efforts. This most likely comes from the WHO focusing on international surveillance and warning, while individual countries are expected to have their own plans in place for dealing with consequences of a pandemic.

- *US Federal Influenza Plans.*[245] In 2005-2006 the White House issued the national pandemic influenza preparedness strategy. In turn HHS issued its plan for pandemic influenza. The 2017 update lists seven domains as a guide for preparedness. These are a set of categories that can guide scenario development for games:

  o Surveillance, Epidemiology, and laboratory activities

  o Community mitigation measures

  o Medical countermeasures (diagnostics, vaccines, therapeutics, and respiratory devices)

  o Health care system preparedness

  o Communications and public outreach

  o Scientific infrastructure and preparedness

  o Domestic and international response policy, incident management and global partnerships

- *Emergency Support Function (ESF) #8 – Public Health and Medical Services Annex.*[246] ESFs are the way the NRF integrates different sets of capabilities and expertise into the IMS. ESF 8 is the medical support function to any sort of disaster. Which can be important if your game is examining a disaster that does not center around disease but one during which disease and injury are part of the disaster and the system has to respond.

- *Biological Incident Annex (BIA) to the Response and Recovery Federal Interagency Operational Plans.*[247] The BIA covers all biological incidents with a branch plan to cover intentional biological events. It covers all types of biological incidents, not just those that create a pandemic. The BIA only

---

[242] Ross (2017) and Adams EH, Scanlon E, Callahan JJ 3rd, Carney MT. (2010) Utilization of an incident command system for a public health threat: West Nile virus in Nassau County, New York, 2008. *J Public Health Manag Pract.* 16(4):309-315. doi:10.1097/PHH.0b013e3181bb8392.

[243] Federal Emergency Management Agency. *National Incident Management System,* October 2017. https://www.fema.gov/media-library/assets/documents/148019

[244] https://www.who.int/influenza/preparedness/pandemic/en/

[245] https://www.cdc.gov/flu/pandemic-resources/planning-preparedness/national-strategy-planning.html

[246] https://www.fema.gov/media-library/assets/documents/25512

[247] Federal Emergency Management Agency. (Jan 2017) *Biological Incident Annex to the Response and Recovery Federal Interagency Operational Plans..* Final.

covers consequence management; law enforcement will have their own plans and processes covering any criminal or national security investigations of the event.

- *HHS and CDC planning.* As the Lead Federal Agency for health response HHS will also have departmental plans for medical and disease events. Most of these plans are managed by the Centers for Disease Control and Prevention (CDC). Plans include:

    o *The National Pandemic Influenza Plan.* This includes the National Strategy for Pandemic Influenza, the corresponding Implementation Plan, and the Departmental (HHS) Influenza Plan.[248]

    o For other diseases, such as Ebola and Zika, CDC planning focused on providing guidelines and recommendations to state and local authorities dealing with the disease.[249]

- *State plans.* States will have their own plans for infectious disease outbreaks or medical events. For example, California has its Infectious Disease Planning Guide, which is a checklist that can be filled out in order to understand preparedness levels.[250] Returning to our example of Florida, that state maintains multiple plans that vary by disease. These range from plans for mosquito-borne disease to legionnaire's disease.[251] These plans are more often framed as guidebooks, training materials, or checklists, but they provide insight into expectations and plans at the state level for when an outbreak occurs. They also inform the plans at the local level by providing the template and training materials for local public health organizations.

- *Local plans.* Cities, counties, and other local governmental entities will have infectious disease emergency response (IDER) plans. Large communities will have more formal, and comprehensive, plans because of their greater resources and requirements. For example, San Francisco has an extensive set of plans.[252]

- *Organizational plans.* In addition to governmental plans, businesses and health care providers may have their own plans. In Florida many licensed health care facilities are required to have Comprehensive Emergency Management Plans (CEMP). These plans are in the form of checklists designed to ensure that risks have been identified and plans for dealing with the risks developed. These forms have to be submitted to the Department of Health.[253]

There are a *lot* of plans, and they extend up and down the chain of command, and across different agencies, localities, and industries. If you are designing a game, they will inform both your design as well as the player actions. For example, with Florida Department of Health requiring a CEMP, many medical organizations will expect to follow their plan – including authorities and regulations – during a game. If, for example, HIPAA (Health Insurance Portability and Accountability Act) regulations prevent the disclosure of the details on areas affected through the release of zip code or other residential information, you may not want to structure the data you give to the players in that way. In fact, that could become a significant issue in the game, with providers having to get rulings, waivers, or exclusions in order to provide HIPAA-controlled data to other health organizations, law enforcement, or the public.

In looking at the plans it is important to understand both what is included, and what is not included. For example, plans may mention HIPAA, health insurance, or liability without going into detail. These issues may actually represent major challenges for the players, and the plans only hint at them mainly because the underlying issues that arise have not yet been resolved through legislation, regulation, or other agreements. These become important components of your scenario and game, because they are the items that often challenge the players the most.

---

[248] https://www.cdc.gov/flu/pandemic-resources/planning-preparedness/national-strategy-planning.html
[249] https://www.cdc.gov/mmwr/volumes/67/wr/mm6735a2.htm and https://www.cdc.gov/vhf/ebola/outbreaks/preparedness/outbreak-preparedness.html
[250] https://emsa.ca.gov/wp-content/uploads/sites/71/2017/07/Infectious-Disease-IPG.pdf
[251] http://www.floridahealth.gov/diseases-and-conditions/index.html
[252] https://www.sfcdcp.org/health-alerts-emergencies/infectious-disease-emergency-response-ider-plan/
[253] https://ahca.myflorida.com/mchq/emergency_activities/index.shtml The emphasis on disaster planning in Florida is likely due to the rather frequent occurrence of major hurricanes and the need to manage patients and residents of health care and assisted living facilities.

Military disease response

There are several components that have to be considered when thinking about the military's role in disease response:

- *Operational defense against biological warfare agents.* The military could, theoretically, encounter biological agents in its mission to defend the country. The organizations charged with preparing and defending against such contingencies have their own organization, plans, and processes.

- *Operational exposure to disease.* More likely than exposure to warfare agents is that forces encounter any number of endemic diseases or wildlife that exist in the area where they are operating. There are military organizations and infrastructure designed to monitor and mitigate the effects of disease on forces. This element is separate from, but overlaps with, organizations responsible for biological defense.

- *Force and family health.* The military provides healthcare for servicemembers and their dependents. It runs hospitals, clinics, and manages the healthcare for a variety of units and organizational elements.

- *Non-military relationships.* The military exists within the context of a community, domestically and overseas. The overall health status of the community can affect base health through support contractors and other personnel brining disease onto the base, aerosol contamination or spread, and through civilian personnel who work as part of units becoming affected off-base and losing productivity. These elements can all affect the military's ability to do its mission, and base commanders have a role to play in coordination with the civilian community, in addition to their military role.

In the US military medicine is a joint enterprise, meaning that it is commanded independently of the services. At the same time the services retain capability and responsibility for the health of their forces and medical support is delivered through service channels. Biological defense of forces is part of the overall Chemical-Biological-Radiological Defense capability and exists as both an agency, the Defense Threat Reduction Agency (DTRA), as well as military units located with the services (examples would be the US Army Chemical Corps or the US Marine Corps Chemical Biological Incident Response Force (CBIRF)).

The corresponding organization charts and roles and responsibilities are too complex to go into here but suffice to say that they are even more byzantine than their civilian counterparts.

When designing a military disease-response game, it is important to ask the following questions:

- *Is the game about disease response in a conflict or "garrison" (peacetime) situation?*
    - If the situation is a conflict, is the problem the result of terrorism, or conventional, large-scale, warfare?
        - If it's terrorism the military will likely be involved either as targets or collateral victims, but the whole unit, installation, or area will be involved in the response. They will need to coordinate with civilian authorities, coordinate medical resources, and implement heightened force protection measures.
        - Terrorism may also imply that Special Operations Forces (SOF) are involved – and may have deliberately or accidentally encountered biological agent. This puts the game down a completely different operational path, in which the game becomes all about the role of the SOF.
        - Biological agents used by enemy forces against US forces in conflict will create a situation in which medical suddenly becomes the central focus for defense of the force. Such use will also raise operational and strategic questions about how the conflict will continue and/ or escalate in the face of the use of disease agents.
    - If it is peacetime or domestic
        - If it's terrorist use then domestic or host nation law enforcement and medical systems will be engaged, and the US military will have a minor supporting role. Military decisions will include force protection, aid to civilian operations, and the ability of various military medical and warfare elements to support consequence-management operations.

- If the disease is naturally occurring, as in the case of a pandemic, then the timelines for response will be longer and the military medical community will be in the lead for detection, prevention, and treatment of the force. This kind of event can become complicated, with trade-offs occurring between force protection, the need to allow personnel on and off base, and the potential exposure of military families.

- *Are the players planning, preparing, or responding?* Planning and preparing for an event allows players to be more fluid in their assumptions about organizational relationships, capabilities, and options. They are writing the script that they will follow during an event. Responding implies that they will have to deal with the threat using what they have, and the relationships and capabilities that currently exist.

- *Is the disease acute or chronic?* This is a question that seldom comes up in military games, because those games are mostly focused on emergency response and consequence management actions. But the role that chronic disease, such as diabetes, heart disease, or traumatic brain injuries play in military medicine is something that could occur as the focus of a game. In addition, because they require resources for treatment, they also affect readiness and force availability. They can also involve the Veteran's Administration, creating seams between organizations where authorities either overlap or are gapped, and issues of authority and responsibility. They can also affect military family members.

The intention in this book is not to detail military disease response operations, particularly biological attack against troops in the field. However, if confronted with the need to do a game on the topic there are several important references to know about,[254] and it will be important to engage with the force surgeon or other military medical personnel to understand the current state of military medicine's organization and capabilities.

Routine disease response

In a routine response operation, the public health community has the lead, and the event is confined to either a small number of dispersed cases, or a larger number of localized cases. Thus the disease response process stays mainly in the public health community, with little spill over into other aspects of disaster response. The interagency process coordinates with public health, but public health has the clear lead.

West Nile Virus is an example of a common, vector-borne disease that the CDC responds to.[255] For West Nile this means that providers report cases to the CDC, and the CDC has to work various issues such as the effect of the disease on the blood supply and how to coordinate across international borders.[256] And West Nile is just one of many diseases that the CDC at least monitors.[257] These types of "routine" disease response operations present an interesting challenge for game design. As the response is ongoing, and will continue after your game, the players will often be familiar with the real-world response. And your game can affect the real-world response. Because of this you have an additional responsibility to get the science, epidemiology, and processes correct. If you don't then your players will likely disengage from the game, or, perhaps worse, learn the wrong lessons.

While these operations may be routine, they also can generate interesting and important questions for the participants

- What constitutes an unusual cluster that is worth responding to?

- How many resources do you devote to a particular situation?

- How will the epidemiologists and medical professionals from all levels of government coordinate their efforts in understanding and managing the cluster of cases?

---

[254] Doctrine, such as Joint Chiefs of Staff (JCS). (11 Dec 2017) Joint Publication 4-02: *Joint Health Services*, is a good place to start but you will need additional information on the service specific organizations and capabilities you will be dealing with. In addition, doctrine on CBR-D can help: JCS (29 Oct 2018) *JP 3-11 Operations in Chemical, Biological, Radiological and Nuclear Environments* and JCS (9 Sep 2016) *JP 3-41 Chemical Biological Radiological and Nuclear Response.* (the effect on capabilities of lumping all of these different things into one family of things is another book.)

[255] Though West Nile was more of a focus when it first came out, it is still one of the overall diseases monitored by the CDC. https://www.cdc.gov/westnile/index.html

[256] https://www.cdc.gov/westnile/statsmaps/index.html

[257] https://wwwn.cdc.gov/nndss/conditions/notifiable/2020/

- How will the public health community interface with the rest of government, and international organizations?

- What public communications should occur related to the operation?

Even for chronic diseases like heart disease, these questions come up, and all may be understood better through gaming.

Zika is an example of a "routine" response that occurred at a large scale. In this case "routine" simply means that there was a large cluster of potential disease cases, and that an organized response occurred within the health community. There was also considerable public pressure to do something about the potential importation of the virus from South America, and the health consequences to pregnant women drove a lot of the concern and interest in the disease.

The Zika virus is also an example of what happens when a routine disease response becomes the focus of the media and the public. In this case because of the potential threat from vector (mosquito) borne transmission in Florida (and potentially elsewhere). In late November 2015 Brazil declared a public health emergency based on the number of Zika cases and reporting that it was associated with microcephaly in newborns and other neurological disorders.[258] And the virus was spreading not only in Brazil but throughout the Central American, Caribbean and South American regions.

After the Pan-American Health Organization (PAHO) published an epidemiological update on Zika in January, 2016 detailing cases of microcephaly, the WHO declared the outbreak a Public Health Emergency of International Concern and the Obama administration moved to increase funding and respond to potential outbreaks within the US. When the funding did not pass Congress, the administration moved other monies to assist in the fight with the disease.

The CDC issued a plan to fight Zika in September 2016 (prior iterations of the plan were circulating well before the official plan was released).[259] The plan defined departmental roles and responsibilities, an action plan, and trigger/decision points. This is effectively an outline for how to build a scenario revolving around a vector borne disease. In reading the plan you will also realize that you need to take into account tribal and territorial governments, particularly Puerto Rico and the US Virgin Islands as they are well within the danger zone for Zika.

Data on the response also highlight a couple of other scenario elements:

- The disease response became politicized, both in terms of how well the response was going and getting the spending bill through Congress.[260] This was a foreshadowing of the political polarization that occurred during the COVID-19 pandemic.[261]

- Communication policy matters in public health events, and it mattered in the Zika response. Studies of risk communications, like the one performed for Zika, can inform game designs by linking player communications actions to media actions and public understandings. For example, the risk-elevating messages in the media during the event may have raised public concerns, placing additional pressure on the public health response.[262]

- The primary and secondary health effects of the virus were evolving. The role that sexual transmission could play was something that arose during the response. The range of possible adverse outcomes was also something that evolved over the course of the event. This, in turn, generated a lot of secondary effects for the CDC and public health authorities, such as developing clinical and public guidelines, testing, length of infectious period and vector control.

- The need to work with local governments on vector control. In the US local governments use an integrated vector management (IVM) plan to control mosquitos. The local mosquito-control

[258] Rasmussen, S. et al. (2016) "Zika Virus and Birth Defects — Reviewing the Evidence for Causality." *N Engl J Med.* 374:1981-1987

[259] Centers for Disease Control and Prevention. (Sep 2016) United States Government Zika Virus Disease Contingency Response Plan.

[260] Harvard T.H. Chan School of Public Health. (Aug 2016) *Zika Virus and the Election Season.*

[261] Seib, G. (18 May 2020) "Why Coronavirus Increasingly Exacerbates the Red-Blue Divide" *Wall St. Journal.*

[262] Sell, T. et al. (2018) "Frequency of Risk-Related News Media Messages in 2016 Coverage of Zika Virus." *Risk Analysis* 38:12:2514-2524.

professionals were needed to survey the local mosquito species in order to understand whether those that spread Zika were present, increase control measures if travel-related infections occurred in their area, and target specific species (*Ades aegypti* and *albopictus*) that transmit the disease. This is an opportunity in a game context to bring in professionals who may not normally participate in games and give the public health professionals an opportunity to coordinate and collaborate with them on vector control.

Chronic, as opposed to acute diseases like Zika, also are a major focus of public health efforts. In all of these games the public health system will work through existing channels and organizations in order to manage the disease outbreak. The emergency response network becomes involved when the risk is to a larger population, or when there is significant political or media focus on the disease. Managing this process of political/social attention against the actual risk from the disease is one of the major challenges that can be incorporated into routine disease-response games.

Pandemic response

For pandemic response, the plans scale up and the interagency process definitely becomes involved. The international community also becomes drawn into plans as one of the definitions of being in a pandemic is that the disease crosses international boundaries.

The definition of a pandemic is: "an epidemic occurring worldwide, or over a very wide area, crossing international boundaries and usually affecting a large number of people."[263] This is a rather loose definition, and subject to interpretation. For example, seasonal outbreaks of the flu are not generally considered pandemics,[264] while a novel flu with a high mortality rate might be, even if it were seasonal.

This alone poses problems for players dealing with a pandemic: when to call it a pandemic and why. There are both disease and political implications. In addition, a "pandemic light" scenario is also completely plausible. For example, the 2009 influenza outbreak,[265] or the 2002-2004 SARs outbreak,[266] were not devastating worldwide, but still required exercising the infrastructure and response plans for pandemics.

For pandemic influenza, the World Health Organization has defined a series of phases for the response.[267] Most of the pandemic phases describe the progress of the virus, not the response. For example, in Pandemic Flu Phase 3 an influenza virus has caused sporadic cases or small clusters of disease in people but has not progressed to human-to-human transmission enough to sustain community-level outbreaks. The focus of the pandemic phases is on whether there is transmission, and how many people will be affected by the transmission. During the period of widespread pandemic transmission (Phase 6 and post-peak) the consequence management phases of the event (closure, partial opening, vaccine production, etc.) are not described.

Within a disease outbreak a lot of things will probably happen, and we can match those events up with the general progress of a disaster response that we discussed in a previous section:[268]

- **Threat identification** (WHO Phases 1-4). The medical and scientific communities have verified that there is a substantial threat from a particular disease outbreak through testing and epidemiology.

- **Threat acceptance** (WHO Phase 5). The political and social communities have accepted that the threat is significant and have begun response operations.

- **Response phase** (WHO Phase 6 – Phase 5 for individual countries or regions). Mitigation efforts are underway through isolation, testing, contact tracing, and medical support to those affected. This phase can have several sub-components including:

    o Containment (isolation, contact tracing, etc.)

---

[263] Last JM, editor. (2001) *A dictionary of epidemiology*, 4th edition.

[264] Heath Kelly. (2011) The classical definition of a pandemic is not elusive *Bulletin of the World Health Organization* 89:540-541. doi: 10.2471/BLT.11.088815

[265] https://www.cdc.gov/flu/pandemic-resources/2009-h1n1-pandemic.html

[266] Knobler S, Mahmoud A, Lemon S, et al., editors. (2004) *Learning from SARS: Preparing for the Next Disease Outbreak: Workshop Summary.* Available from: https://www.ncbi.nlm.nih.gov/books/NBK92467/

[267] World Health Organization. (2017) *WHO Pandemic Phase Descriptions and Main Actions by Phase.* Undated.

[268] This is a different version of what can be found in Rose.

- Laboratory (typing, testing for resistance, developing probes, DNA sequencing)

- Treatment (vaccine and medicinal development including prophylaxis)

- Medical (providing care for patients)

- Certifications, regulations, and standards (FDA approval of tests/treatments, standards for cleanliness, etc.)

- Mortuary

- Mitigation (cleaning and disinfecting contaminated areas)[269]

- Infrastructure (sustainment of critical infrastructure and capabilities)

- Informatics (managing data, scientific, and response information surrounding the event)

- Information (messaging and public information)

- **Recovery phase** (WHO Post-Peak Period). During this phase the containment measures are slowly relaxed prior to an effective treatment or the seasonal variation in disease cases. This phase can cycle several times as follow-on waves of disease arrive either because of seasonal variations or because of relaxed mitigation measures.

- **Treatment phase** (WHO Post-Peak Period). An effective treatment has been developed; now it has to be produced, allocated to various populations, and distributed. This can run simultaneously with the recovery and response phases if a treatment already exists for the disease.

- **Threat monitoring** (WHO Post-Pandemic Period). This is the ongoing monitoring that occurs in order to identify and recognize emerging threats. In the case of terrorism, it represents the deployment of sensors, law enforcement and military actions, pre-staging of prophylaxis and treatment supplies.

For pandemics the monitoring and detection phase is never really over. This is equivalent to the mitigation phase in a disaster response framework. Monitoring is also sufficiently complex that the WHO breaks it down into different phases. This means that for games on pandemics it's important to understand what phase you are in, and what you are trying to simulate. Figure 4 shows a timeline using the WHO phases, with additional consequence management phases superimposed over them.

You can put on pandemic games that involve any of the response phases:

- *Disease surveillance, detection, identification, and notification (Phases 1-2).* Here games could range from a focus on field work, sample collection, transportation, and processing to ones involving laboratory capacity and building long-term international surveillance. This would be quite suitable for a board game, with the geography of the area of interest represented by the board and players representing local public health, international epidemiologists, and institutional (laboratory) managers. The players would be allocating assets, managing samples and sample biosecurity, and applying different techniques and technologies to analyzing the data that they were collecting. So, if they fund a trip to the bat caves to collect and return samples, they have to allocate both zoonotic expertise, sample collection equipment, biosecurity professionals, and transport. These will be unusable for the duration of the expedition. There will be a payoff for a successful expedition, likely the ability to more easily detect the next zoonotic outbreak that occurs as a result of having more PCR/ELISA probes.

- *Alert process (Phases 3-4).* During pandemic stages 3 and 4 a virus has been identified as circulating in the human population. However, it has not broken out into large population groups yet. In this game the emphasis will be on detection, notifications, threat assessment, initial mitigation actions, and preparation. The index government will have the choice of doing nothing, decreasing exposure, or preparing for a potential pandemic by stockpiling resources and communicating the threat. Games at this level will naturally focus on the interface between public health, government decision-making, and politics. To follow-on with the above zoonotic case, we now have the first human-to-human

---

[269] For example, there were issues with cleaning buildings after the 2001 anthrax attacks, particularly the American Media International building in Boca Raton, Florida. National Research Council. (2005) *Reopening Public Facilities After a Biological Attack: A Decision Making Framework.* Washington, DC: The National Academies Press. https://doi.org/10.17226/11324.

transmission occurring in our country's population. It is likely the disease migrated from bats to a mammal and then to humans. Initially the players know nothing about what is going on. They have their normal resources and have to allocate them against potential collection targets (zoonotic, laboratory monitoring, hospitals, database analysis,[270] etc.). Once detected then they can make the case for more resources, or various social solutions to the problem.

- *Pandemic games (Phase 5-6 and Post Pandemic).* This is what we normally think of when we think of a pandemic game. Here the focus is on mitigating the effects of the virus, managing medical resources, and dealing with other consequences of the pandemic. That is why I overlapped the traditional emergency response functions over these phases. During these phases governments and the international community have made a decision to take decisive action. But these actions may be affected by political considerations, and information about the pandemic may change some of the approaches taken. In this game you have an uncontained outbreak, you are using the SIR model to project infection rates, and the players have all elements of national power, constrained by political and social considerations, to use against the outbreak.

In a pandemic game the characteristics of the disease will play a major role in determining how, exactly, the pandemic phase will go. The type of consequence management, and the nature of the medical response will depend on the nuanced details of the disease. Fortunately, as you can see from the ongoing COVID-19 pandemic, even after six months or more of intense research there are many factors about the disease that are still unknown, unresolved, or variable. For example, the role of demographics in determining infectivity of those with the virus. The notion of "superspreaders" or superspreader events in which large numbers of individuals are infected by one individual. These and other parameters are not well understood, even well into the pandemic. This gives the game designer a lot of room to manage the game through managing the biology of the disease.

---

[270] For example, there are many schemes to monitor public data in order to detect outbreaks: Pivette, Mathilde et al. (18 Nov 2014) "Drug sales data analysis for outbreak detection of infectious diseases: a systematic literature review." *BMC infectious diseases* vol. 14 604. doi:10.1186/s12879-014-0604-2

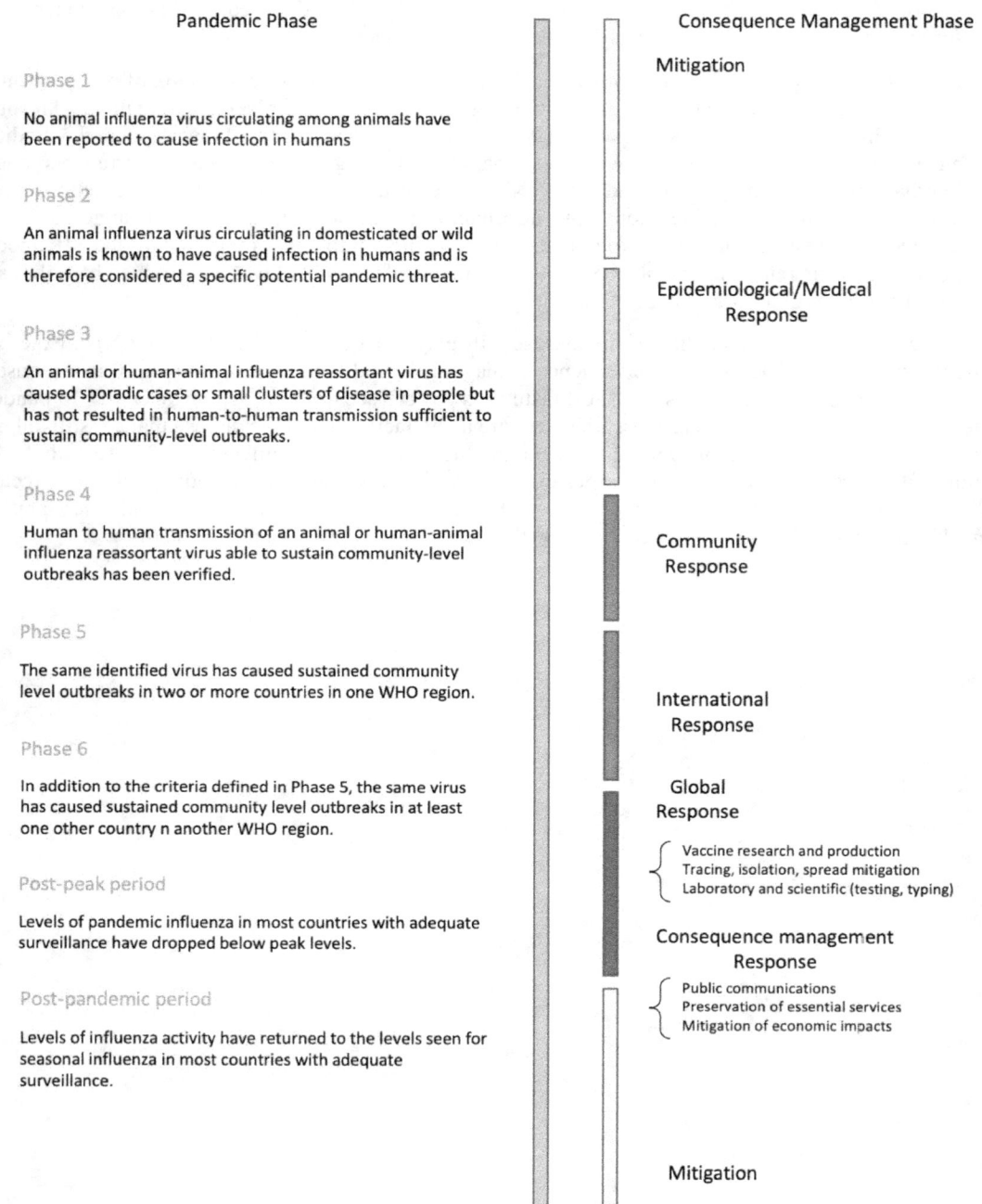

Pandemic Phase

Phase 1

No animal influenza virus circulating among animals have been reported to cause infection in humans

Phase 2

An animal influenza virus circulating in domesticated or wild animals is known to have caused infection in humans and is therefore considered a specific potential pandemic threat.

Phase 3

An animal or human-animal influenza reassortant virus has caused sporadic cases or small clusters of disease in people but has not resulted in human-to-human transmission sufficient to sustain community-level outbreaks.

Phase 4

Human to human transmission of an animal or human-animal influenza reassortant virus able to sustain community-level outbreaks has been verified.

Phase 5

The same identified virus has caused sustained community level outbreaks in two or more countries in one WHO region.

Phase 6

In addition to the criteria defined in Phase 5, the same virus has caused sustained community level outbreaks in at least one other country n another WHO region.

Post-peak period

Levels of pandemic influenza in most countries with adequate surveillance have dropped below peak levels.

Post-pandemic period

Levels of influenza activity have returned to the levels seen for seasonal influenza in most countries with adequate surveillance.

Consequence Management Phase

Mitigation

Epidemiological/Medical Response

Community Response

International Response

Global Response
{ Vaccine research and production
Tracing, isolation, spread mitigation
Laboratory and scientific (testing, typing)

Consequence management Response
{ Public communications
Preservation of essential services
Mitigation of economic impacts

Mitigation

Figure 4 – WHO Pandemic Phases and disaster phases[271]

For a pandemic disease the parameters that matter most, and coincidently the parameters that are often the least understood, include:

---

[271] World Health Organization (undated) *WHO Pandemic Phase Descriptions and Main Actions by Phase.*

- *Transmissibility.* How easily does the disease transmit from one individual to another? Transmissibility of the influenza virus can be broken down into:
  - *Exposure to particles.* This is inhalation of either tiny nano particles (<5 microns) or bulk droplets. Particles can also lodge in other mucus membranes and potentially represent an infection pathway.
  - *Contact.* Contact with fomites, or a contaminated surface, and then contact with mucus membranes like your nose, eyes, or mouth can also result in transmission.
  - *Uncommon.* Fecal-oral is one route. Which has gotten some publicity in recent days due to the possibility of COVID-19 being transmitted through aerosols generated by flushing toilets.[272] Animal vectors are another possible route.

Other parameters that are important include:

- *Infectious period.* How long are patients "effectively" infectious for? Some patients may be highly infectious, but lack the ability to move about and infect others. Other patients may be highly infectious and show no symptoms, allowing them to spread the disease far and wide. Asymptomatic or pre-symptomatic spread is the game designer's best friend, because is subverts many of the typical limiting factors on disease transmission.

- *Lethality.* Lethality by age (or other demographic cohort) is especially important because of the different roles that children, adults, and the elderly play in a disease response. A disease that is highly lethal in children will require a significantly different response than one that only affects the elderly.

- *Survivability in the environment.* Not only is the overall survivability of the disease a concern, but the locations where it can survive is also important. A virus that is survivable in water (unlikely for flu) will pose a very different set of challenges than one which is easily washed away.

- *Disease progression.* As we saw with Melioidosis not all diseases are over after an infection occurs. In some cases, they can have longer-term effects, affecting different organs or have fetal or natal effects, like Zika. Likelihood of sepsis and septic shock, along with the occurrence of pneumonias are also important parameters.

- *Immune response.* There are at least three factors that matter for games:
  - Effect on immune-compromised individuals
  - Likelihood of a cytokine storm occurring (over-active immune response)
  - Duration and strength of immunity from having the disease, or from immunization.

- *Immunization and treatment.* The susceptibility of the disease to immunization and treatment is another parameter. A disease that is not easily immunized for (think common cold) will be harder to deal with than one where a vaccine is stable and highly effective (seasonal flu). Lack of treatment options will also increase the overall lethality of the agent.

While these routes may seem relatively straightforward to model, the details and dynamics are actually quite complex. For example, with the aerosol spread the effective dose may not be well understood, and the interaction of the virus with the environment may be unknown. Thus, a situation where an individual is exposed to a low dose outside in sunlight may have dramatically different effects than a high viral-load exposure inside a contained area. These dynamics are often lost in the rolling up of the overall parameters for population models, which we have discussed before.

In a game design we are not just concerned with overall population effects of the disease. As is the case with COVID-19, decision-makers need additional data beyond basic reproduction rate in order to make informed decisions about prevention and response. A disease that is survivable in high humidity, high temperature, and exposure to UV will be more of a threat in the summer than a disease with those as limiting factors. A disease that is highly survivable on surfaces, and infectious in low doses will be a bigger threat than one with only moderate survivability.

---

[272] Wang, Ji-Xiang, et al. (2020) "Can a toilet promote virus transmission? From a fluid dynamics perspective," *Physics of Fluids* **32**, 065107; https://doi.org/10.1063/5.0013318

Note that none of these parameters includes the origin of the disease. In some cases, this may become important (when zoonotic vectors are considered) in controlling the outbreak. There also may be political reasons to understand the origin, for assigning blame or attribution[273].

The sheer variety of parameters, and the combinations they produce, give the game designer a lot of latitude in designing a pandemic disease. COVID-19 has a parameter set that, if included in a game, would create a lot of skepticism amongst the players that the game designer was stacking the deck against them. It is highly transmissible, survives in the summer, and is asymptomatically spread. The only thing players in a COVID-19 game would have going for them is its lethality-age curve with older demographics being hit harder than younger ones. Higher lethality in younger demographics would result in a much more difficult set of choices in how to respond to the disease.

Asymptomatic spread, along with high lethality in younger demographics, are examples of parameters that the game designer can use to adjust the degree of difficulty and political concern.

The number of people and the demographics of those affected by a disease are tools in the designer's toolbox that tells government and public health players how well they are doing with respect to disease control. Other factors, such as lethality, modes of transmission, and effectiveness of treatment tell the public health and government players what they need to do to limit transmission of the disease and change the numbers. A disease that spreads only in symptomatic patients, and only with high viral dose loads, will tend to respond well to aggressive contact tracing. A disease that spreads asymptomatically at low viral loads may require whole-of-population measures (movement controls and restrictions, masking, etc.) in order to control its spread.

As we discussed in previous chapters all of these parameters are related to the number of infected through the basic reproduction number and the SIR equations. But even with the same R_0 two agents with radically different sets of parameters will require different kinds of response and involve different agencies and capabilities. A disease that is very survivable in the environment may engage the Environmental Protection Agency (EPA) and others who have experience decontaminating difficult agents. A disease that transmits through nanoparticles in the environment will engage those experienced with air handling and fluids.

This means that the disease parameters are tools that you can use in a pandemic game to stress and explore the game objectives. A game in which movement control implementation and effects are important may require a virus that spreads asymptomatically, or at least pre-symptomatically. A game in which the fate of the agent in the environment, and in which decontamination is important would have a biochemistry that rendered it highly survivable in the environment and on surfaces.

Pandemic games are driven by the characteristics of the disease, but the disease drives a complex set of medical, disaster response, and political decisions.

Non-infectious disease response

Games on non-infectious disease are not in as much demand as those dealing with infectious disease. Non-infectious diseases include chronic diseases like heart disease and diabetes, as well as accidents and trauma injuries. Examples of possible non-infectious disease games include:

- Games looking at interagency coordination, and public-private partnerships, to address lifestyle choices on chronic disease. Questions could include how public information campaigns could coordinate with PVO/NGO efforts to reduce the incidence of various chronic diseases. In the US, health insurance companies also play a role in shaping response to chronic diseases. Since the information campaign is an integral part of responding to chronic diseases the insurance industry may have a role in integrating into those actions.

- An emergency room game to examine resource allocation, patient flow, timing and cost of ER visits. While emergency-room flow can be understood through analysis,[274] many of the human and organizational factors that go into ER operations can affect outcomes. Understanding how nurses,

---

[273] Consider the naming of Spanish Flu in 1918/19 and the continuing attempts to divert attention from the origins of Covid 19 in 2020/21.

[274] Miró, O et al. (2003) "Analysis of patient flow in the emergency department and the effect of an extensive reorganisation." *Emergency Medicine Journal : EMJ* vol. 20,2 143-8; discussion 148. doi:10.1136/emj.20.2.143

support staff, administrative hospital staff, doctors and patients all approach their roles in the ER may identify areas that analysis might miss in optimizing variables in the ER.

- A game representing the management of blood-borne diseases and how public health, blood supply, and medical systems can coordinate against a potential long-term threat to the blood supply. This would draw on experiences with AIDS, COVID-19, and others to explore an emerging threat to the ability to collect, manage, and allocate blood within the medical system.

- A game to explore changes to the process and laws surrounding compensation for organ and tissue donation. Currently the system is largely supplied with organs and other supplies through donation. There is an ongoing debate about whether organ donors should somehow be compensated in order to induce donation, either posthumously or while alive.[275] A game could bring together the different viewpoints, and put them into an implementation scenario where all of the issues could be discussed and evaluated from the perspective of making it work (or not).

Non-infectious disease games almost always center around political, policy, or interagency questions because response is slow and longer term. However just because a response is slow does not mean that many of the same issues seen in rapid-onset responses don't occur. They just evolve more slowly over time, giving responders more time to evaluate options. When considering a game like this the management of time relative to player decisions becomes even more important than it does in rapid-response games.

In almost any game players can legitimately argue that they would have more time to develop courses of action, evaluate data, and make decisions than they are given in the game. For rapid-response games the reply is that, while you might have three hours in the real world instead of the one you have in the game, most of those three hours would be spent answering e-mail, orienting yourself to the problem, or on other overhead duties. The actual time for decisions might be less than you are given in the game.

In a slow-onset game this will not be the case. Players can argue that decisions are spread over days or even years. However, it is often not the details of the response or data that drive decisions in slow-onset disease responses, but rather the politics of the situation. It may be easy to prove that paying top dollar for organs brings out the donors, but that data is easily overruled by the potential social and political arguments.

Non-infectious disease games will:

- *Have turns that represent long periods of time.* Each move may be months or even years so that interventions and decisions can play out in the populations. This requires the game designers to build scenarios that incorporate confounding and supporting variables that may have nothing to do with player actions. For example, a trend toward unsweetened drinks in consumer preferences as a trend that reduces obesity.

- *Require feedback on in game research.* In these games the designers and controllers will need to give dynamic feedback to the players on research questions. For example, in a game on lung cancer, there will be epidemiological research required to understand the disease, and laboratory research to develop treatments and vaccines. These will need to both conform to the game objectives, and tie player investment decisions to outcomes. If players conduct research focused on cities, it may be that pollution is found to be a potential cause of higher rates of some lung cancers. Control may need details on the mechanism, the affected populations, and the concentration levels that trigger higher incidences of the cancers. If players then choose to invest in genetic treatments to support a particularly vulnerable population, control will need to be able to relate the cost of that research to a timeline, and potential outcomes.

- *Allow for disease dynamics.* Epidemiological reporting from hospitals and the public health community will generate a considerable amount of baseline data for the disease. Updating those baselines according to player actions will be the responsibility of game control. Often control will be presented with player actions that affect the epidemiological data in ways that are difficult to predict. Some options include:
    - *Use data for similar diseases or treatments.* For example, if a new lung cancer chemotherapy takes 2 years to develop and the roll out takes 1 year with a 10% change in overall survival

---

[275] Harbell, Jack W.; Mathur, Amit K. (Apr 2019) Financial compensation for organ donors, *Current Opinion in Organ Transplantation*: Volume 24 - Issue 2 - p 182-187 doi: 10.1097/MOT.0000000000000617

rates, then the genetic therapy mentioned previously might follow a similar path with some variation. The key is to give the players a "close enough" result that is believable and within the range of variance they would expect in the real world.

- o *Work the process.* Most treatments and other medical actions have to go through some sort of process. First, they have to be developed, then the Food and Drug Administration has to approve them for testing, they have to be tested, data must be collected and analyzed, then the data must be reviewed. This is followed by production and distribution of the treatment. These processes, at least for ordinary, non-infectious diseases, are fairly standard and the times can be deduced from experience and the literature.

- o *Use game objectives.* In a game with specific goals, say to understand mitigation measures in the case of lung cancer, the objective of the game requires players to deal with the topic. They cannot simply take any action that they might want to, rather it has to be related to the game objective. In such a game, control adjusts the outcomes and timings of events to focus the players on game objectives.[276] In games where the objective requires players to pass certain decision points, this is perfectly fine as long as the values used by control do not deviate excessively from the expected variance.

- • *Require some public, policy, and political inputs.* This means that some roles in the game will be political or policy roles. These could represent health system (insurance, hospitals), governmental, or non-governmental organizations. Non-governmental and political players will also need feedback, support, and input from the public's interest and concern in the disease. It is often difficult for professionals, like medical or epidemiological professionals, to play the role of political operatives or non-medical officials. That is because there are other variables that need to be taken into account in political and policy decisions than just the possible patient outcomes. Having players with political— or at least little medical—experience in these roles can be important for generating realistic outcomes in the games.

Games on non-infectious diseases are a three-way challenge: responding to the public's interest or concern, developing the medical and epidemiological response, and managing the policy and political aspects of any response. In order to accomplish this, control will need to incorporate political play, build reasonable and flexible models of timing, cost, and effects, as well as incorporate media and public points of view.

---

[276] This is called inductive game control, where the topic is not open-ended but rather the game needs to progress toward a specific objective in order to be successful.

Chapter 16: Outbreak Investigation

The time is: 0900 EDT. July 11. Virginia Department of Health.

The Director's morning briefing was going fine, until he noticed the large number of reported pneumonias in Loudon and Fairfax Counties, Virginia. There were reports that at least on child had died, and several others were suffering from serious respiratory distress in hospitals in the two counties. Already the parents of the fatality were on the local news: "A child has died of a mysterious respiratory illness. It came on suddenly, no one has any answers, why don't people have answers?" Even if he didn't think it was unusual, the CDC would, and would be calling pretty soon. He decided to dispatch a couple of his public health officers over to Fairfax and Loudon Inova to see what was going on. He also picked up the phone to call the school commissioner. At least DHS had not noticed, yet. Today was not starting off very well.

Objective

Not all disease outbreaks result in thousands of cases and hundreds of deaths. Some are just simple outbreaks that the public health service has to investigate, and deal with on a routine basis. This game seeks to exercise the federal, state, and local disease monitoring, reporting, and analyses processes in a situation of some urgency, and much ambiguity. The sponsor might be the Virginia Department of Health (VDH), the CDC as part of a training program for local public health systems, or HHS headquarters to better understand early-phase outbreaks and local epidemiological plans and processes. The primary objective is: how does the system that is in place differentiate between a major outbreak, terrorism, and a minor outbreak? A secondary objective is to help build interdepartmental coordination between health, fish and wildlife, and regulatory bodies in Virginia. In this case the agency that regulates summer camps.[277]

Background

Hantavirus Pulmonary Syndrome is a disease caused by the Hantavirus, a hemorrhagic fever spread by rodents and endemic to North America. In North America Hantavirus causes hantavirus pulmonary syndrome (HPS) which affects between 24 to 40 people each year, mostly in the Southwest. While cases are centered in the Southwest they have occurred in many different states within the US. The cases we are going to focus on are those that occurred in Virginia in 2004.[278]

Hantavirus is rare in the Eastern United States, but cases of the Monongahela hantavirus strain have occurred there, including our cases in Virginia. In Virginia the virus is transmitted by the white footed mouse and contracted from close contact with the mouse droppings or other aerosolized infectious material. In order to get infected it appears that the exposure must be both prolonged and substantial. In the 2004 Virginia outbreak one individual was a graduate student working with wild rodents and the other had cleaned a cabin infested with mice.

There has, however, been a report of HPS being transmitted between persons in Peru.[279]

The onset of HPS is rapid, within days. The symptoms of HPS are fever, soreness, headache, nausea, vomiting, abdominal pain, and coughing. Within 3-6 days the disease progresses with coughing, shortness of breath, fever and hypotension. Fluid on the lungs (pulmonary edema) occurs and requires ventilation. For HPS the primary cause of death is lung failure. Once the disease passes, recovery is rapid, so the patients should not have long hospital stays.[280]

The fatality rate is 35-45%. The treatment is respiratory management, and drugs to prevent toxic shock. Death in cases of *H. Monongahela* from Pennsylvania and Virginia occurred between 3 and 5 days after onset.[281] This

---

[277] In Virginia it is the Virginia Office of Environmental Health Services under the Virginia Department of Health. https://www.vdh.virginia.gov/environmental-health/

[278] Centers for Disease Control and Prevention. (26 Nov 2004) "Two Cases of Hantavirus Pulmonary Syndrome — Randolph County, West Virginia, July 2004". *MMWR*. 53:46:1083 - 1102

[279] Wells, R. et al. (Apr-Jun 1997) *Emerging Infectious Diseases: Dispatches*. 3:2:171-174

[280] Escutanaire (2000)

[281] Georgia Department of Health. Hantavirus Pulmonary Syndrome (HPS): Fact Sheet. And Rhodes, L. et al. (Nov-Dec 2000) "Hantavirus Pulmonary Syndrome Associated with Monongahela Virus, Pennsylvania," *Emerging Infectious Diseases*. 6:6. Pp 616-621.

is faster than associated with other forms of the disease and may be related to viral dosage. In this scenario I'm going to assume a 3-5 day incubation period with a rapid onset and death within 3-5 days of symptom onset.

Because these incidents were closely associated with cabins and wilderness locations our initial vector will be white-footed-mice infestations in cabins and old buildings near a campsite. This will give us the opportunity for a significant exposure, but through a natural mechanism. The progression of the disease will take full advantage of the six-week time limit on developing symptoms, allowing us to have a strong initial signal and then let the follow-on cases play out in the community.

The setting will be the fictional SunnyTree Overnight Camp located in a rural area of Loudon County, Virginia. Figure 5 shows the counties in Northern Virginia and the relative locations mentioned here.

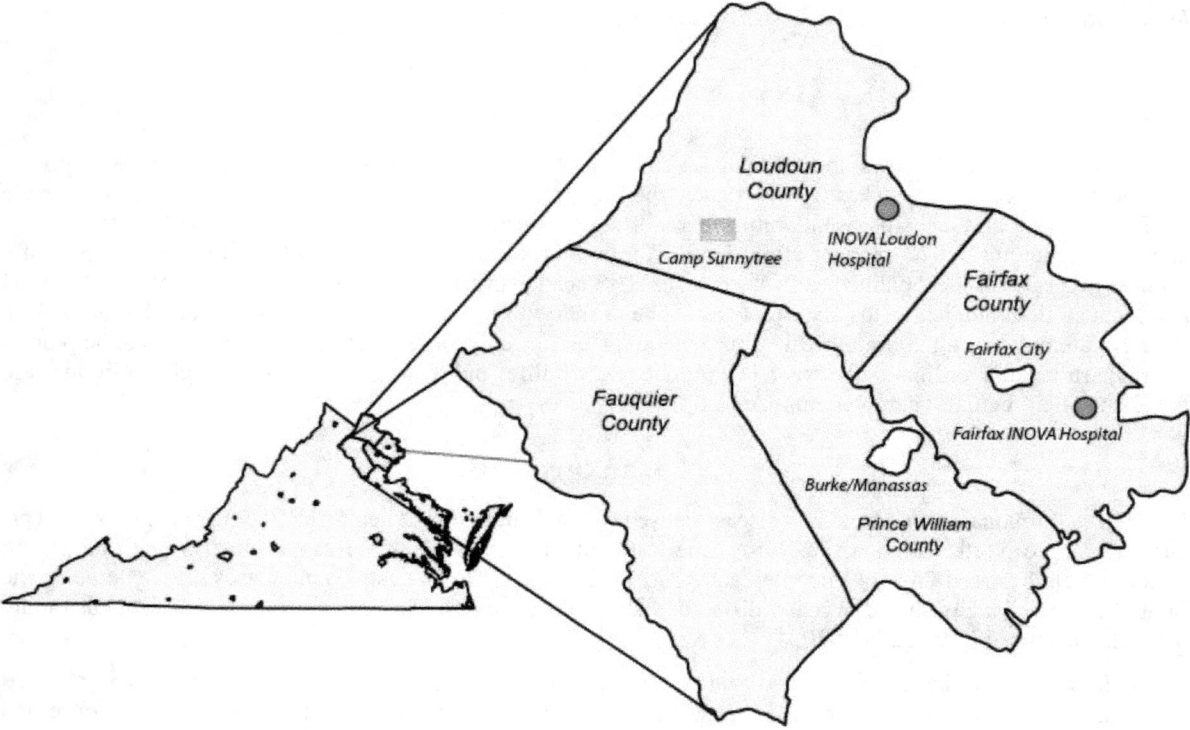

Figure 5 – Northern Virginia

This camp has summer programs for both day and overnight campers. Most of the overnight campers come for 2-3 nights, but other stay for a week or more. Most overnight campers come from Fairfax County, while day campers come primarily from the more suburban areas of Loudon County. The camp is divided up into a central recreation and administrative area, with cabins strung out along a small river. There is an old farm across the river and up an embankment. The farm is dilapidated and run down, but it is a favorite illicit hangout for the campers. In back of the farm the ground rises steeply up to the summit of Bald Tree Mountain.

Figure 6 shows the layout of the camp.

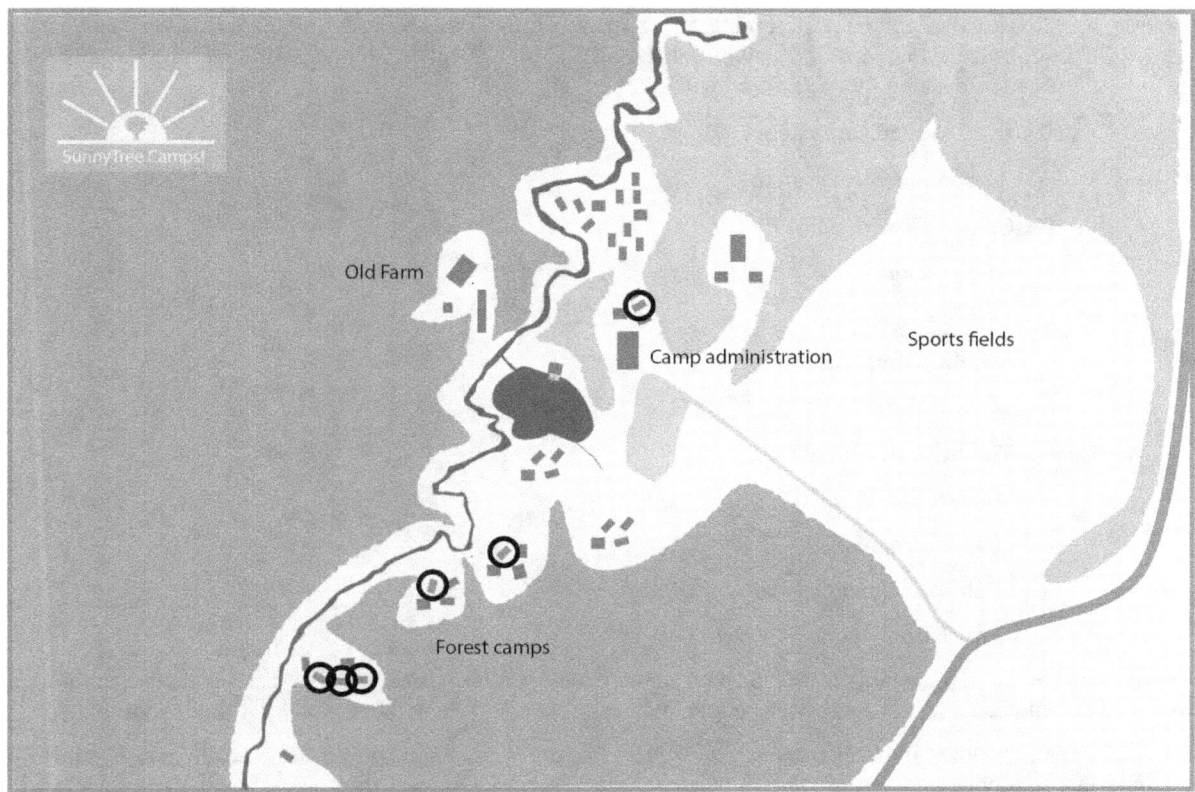

Figure 6 – Layout of SunnyTree Camp with Hantavirus positive cabins are circled.

As you can see in the figure above, we've created a set of old farm buildings, and several campsites out in the woods. This gives us options to have campers exposed in their cabins, or when they go to the Old Farm. This allows some cabins not in the woods to have cases as well, complicating the epidemiology slightly.

Players

The game is designed for a state or local public health service. It could, however, be played with students or others but the level of background information would need to increase. The loss of any medical or public health subject matter experts would require the addition of considerable learning materials, likely to include videos on public health response and epidemiological tracing.

Primary player roles are:

- Virginia Department of Health, Office of Epidemiology
- Loudon County Health Department
    - Director
    - Epidemiologist
    - Laboratory Services
- Fairfax County Health Department
    - Director
    - Epidemiologist
    - Laboratory Services
- Virginia Department of Wildlife Resources (DWR)

- CDC/National Center for Emerging and Zoonotic Infectious Diseases (NCEZID)/Division of High-Consequence Pathogens and Pathology (DHCPP)/Viral Special Pathogens Branch[282] (i.e., where the notification through the NNDSS[283] will land).

- Fairfax INOVA medical system

- INOVA Loudon medical system

- Fairfax County Government

  o Supervisor

  o School Board

  o Public Communications

  o Law enforcement

- Loudon County Government

  o Supervisor

  o School Board

  o Public Communications

  o Law enforcement

These roles can be populated as teams, or with individuals. We have broken down task elements within each role to accommodate a larger number of people, but each role could easily be played by a single individual.

The game spans both the medical response, as well as the governmental response. The health care system will be important to identifying and treating the disease, the CDC, VDOH, and the county health departments will need to identify the location of the outbreak and the potential cause, and the various governments will need to develop advisories regarding the outbreak, and provide assistance to the epidemiologists as they investigate.

Another aspect of this game that we did not emphasize, but could be incorporated, is the role of the Federal and State Departments of Homeland Security and Law Enforcement Agencies. An unknown respiratory condition presenting in a significant number of children may raise the alarm bells about possible terrorist use of agent and warrant the initiation of a counter-terrorism investigation. We decided not to go there, but it would be a logical outcome of the outbreak. You would need to modify the presentation of the cases a little bit in order to encourage this line of investigation, and you may want to put some suspects in the area to give the LEA something to chase. This would exercise coordination between Federal, State, and local LEA along with coordination with Public Health.

Game Concept

The game begins on day six, with day zero being the initial exposure to the virus. It will be important to keep a timeline to ensure we are within parameters for the progression of the disease. All individuals are between the ages of 9 and 12 years old and have attended the SunnyTree Camp either as day or overnight campers. None of this is known to the players at the beginning of the game. Presentations occur to the various hospital systems, who then must act.

Note that the timeline and nature of the presentations of the disease will drive the scenario. We can drive it toward a terrorist concern by placing the worst cases first in a cluster, or we can build public concern by dribbling out cases the way we are doing. Once the source of the disease is discovered, another couple of cases presenting will undermine the public health narrative that things are under control, requiring more public communications and work with the state and local governments.

At the beginning of the game, we will have the following ground truth:

---

[282] https://www.cdc.gov/ncezid/who-we-are/org-ncezid.html
[283] NNDSS: National Notifiable Diseases Surveillance System. The public health surveillance system for the CDC. https://wwwn.cdc.gov/nndss/data-collection.html

- Approximately six days ago five campers spent several hours investigating the old farmhouse and chicken coop. They did not realize that it was an old chicken coop and stirred up considerable dust. These individuals are spread evenly amongst the affected cabins. They will present according to the following timeline:

    o Male, age 9: presents Day 3 to Fairfax: Septic; dies Day 5: Diagnosis Day 6

    o Male age 10, Female Age 11: present Day 4 to Loudon: Condition deteriorating day 6: No diagnosis

    o Female age 10: presents on Day 7 to Fairfax: Succumbs to pneumonia Day 10: Diagnosis depends on events

    o Male age 12: presents on Day 8 Loudon: Begins recovery on Day 11: No diagnosis

- Over the course of the past two weeks several individuals have been exposed in the Forest Camps to low level infectious doses of Hanta by a mouse infestation. They will present according to the following timeline:

    o Male age 9 : presented day 1 to Loudon: remains hospitalized: Diagnosis depends on events

    o Female age 11 and Female age 10: presented day 4 to Fairfax: 1 dies from pneumonia Day 6, 1 recovering Day 6: Diagnosis Day 6

    o Male age 10 and Male age 10: present on Day 8 Fairfax both develop pneumonia and are recovering: Diagnosis depends on events

    o Female age 12: presents on Day 9 Loudon with severe pneumonia : Dies Day 10 : Diagnosis depends on events

    o Female age 3 (sister to 11 year old Fairfax patient that presented on day 4): presents day 6 to Fairfax : succumbs to pneumonia on day 10 : Diagnosis depends on events

On Day 6 both hospital systems will notice an uptick in unknown respiratory conditions in 9-12 year old children, especially after the fatality. The mom of the fatality will contact local media and begin to raise alarms about potential disease exposure.

The presentation of the disease should be adapted to the overall objectives of the game. Here I've focused on public communications and how the presentations will be seen by the public. You will need to flesh in the addresses and other details for all the individuals. It is important to make sure that you create fictional individuals in order to avoid liability issues. Epidemiologists will want to know where they live, where they have travelled, and where they go to school.

The inclusion of the younger sister of one of the victims is designed to increase epidemiological complexity, this is a rare case of human-to-human transmission but in designing the scenario you can assume that there will be a lot of player focus on that individual because they are anomalous. This will require you to provide a lot of additional detail given that the presumption will be that she contracted it from her sister. Given that human to human transmission is rare it is likely they will want a full traceout on that individual.

The game will not be a long or complex one. The initial presentation will occur to the two hospital systems, who will have 3 days to report it up to the VDOH.[284] Once its reported to the state and county it will be up to the state to coordinate the responses between the counties. The deployment of investigators will need to occur; with a sufficiently large outbreak there will need to be more than one site to be examined. We have included the DWR in the list of players in case they play a role in trapping or hunting wildlife to test for animal cases.

Some things to take into account about environmental testing:

- The actual Virginia cases of HPS were reported in July, the environmental assessment occurred in August.

---

[284] Virginia Department of Health. (Nov 2018) *Virginia Reportable Disease List.*

- In the Virginia case all locations were tested, and the nucleic acid sequences were found to be identical between rodents collected from the two locations (patient A and B). The sequences from the rodents were similar, but not identical, to those in patient A.[285]

- In another case located in Pennsylvania approximately 50% of the mice trapped at the various locations for the two patients had antibodies to the Monongahela virus. The sequences were again identical.

This suggests that environmental sampling in the game should give a hit for positive antibody/virus tests of between 20 and 50% depending on the location. This will depend on player actions. If the players engage the DWR then their expertise may increase the overall collection success rate, and if they tests both sites with multiple traps then that may also increase success rate. Remember the actual infestations are in the forest cabins and the old farm, traps in other areas may catch mice but they will have a much lower chance of being infected.

The cooperation of the camp should be almost assured, because otherwise they could lose their permit to operate. However, their legal and public relations teams will want to minimize the impact of any public communications on the camp.

Questions for the players include:

- How does the notification system operate? Prior to diagnosis of HPS all the hospitals have is an unusual outbreak of pneumonia amongst several children. How do the hospitals communicate on disease? Will they be able to identify the trend prior to the diagnosis? How will diagnosis in one facility be transmitted to the other facilities (remember the reporting requirement is up the chain, not across)? In other words, how will this work exactly, and what will the timeline be? By the time it gets disseminated all of the cases could be in play, the parents could be up in arms, and the situation easily could go out of control. Be prepared for this as the controller.

- What is your public communications strategy? What are you going to tell the public, when, and how? What can you not tell the public for legal reasons? What about the rare case of person-to-person transmission? How will that be presented to the public?

- What will local authorities be concerned about? What happens if the media make the association of HPS with "hemorrhagic fever"? How will the outbreak of a "hemorrhagic fever" in children affect policy and school board actions?

  o This is the least likely area for action: "we don't care" is always a possibility for players as a course of action, although a very dull one. At that point you can increase parental pressure and media attention. But you should be prepared to focus on this if you include governmental players in the game.

- How will the CDC, VDH, and local public health authorities react? What will happen? Will teams be deployed? What will they do?

- How will the epidemiologists (assuming they are deployed) deal with the 3-year-old patient?

- What is the role of the communities involved? Will the Louden Sheriff close off the camp? How will that be enforced? What about the old farm?

- How will the farm and camp be certified as disease free? What will happen if the agencies cannot certify them? Who will enforce closure until certification occurs?

- White footed mice are endemic to the region; what are public health officials going to do to make sure this doesn't happen at other camps.

I could continue to provide additional detail as the game builds out, but that will very much depend on the exact objectives, the player roles, the number of players, and your own point of view.

Execution

The way in which the disease will present suggests a highly structured seminar game, with turns carefully defined based on the timing of the presentations.

---

[285] CDC (2004).

The game should begin with an orientation to the game environment, and to the scenario. Players will likely be unfamiliar with what is about to happen, so it is better if control walks them through the process of how to play the game in some detail. Likewise, they may, or may not, be familiar with hantavirus. Or some of them may have dealt with the monongahela strain before. In the process of designing the game and recruiting the players control/design should talk to some of the players who might have participated in past responses and understand what their knowledge base is. It is far more effective, both in terms of gameplay and in terms of information uptake, for a participant/player to brief the other players on the disease than control. If there are players with monongahela experience then one possible path is for control to not even disclose the disease up front, relying on knowledgeable players to bring the other players up to speed the way they would in the real world. This also has the benefit of giving an important role to the knowledgeable players, which increases the play experience and acceptance of the game.

Turn 1

I would begin the game on Day 6. We have at least four presentations of the disease, which means that someone might notice. Certainly, some of the parents may have contacted the media. I would give the information to the medical players at the very start of the game, so they would have already made their decisions when Turn 1 starts. This way all the other players aren't sitting around waiting for something to happen.

This is a very important, but tricky, part of the game. The players know they are in a disease response game, so the minute you give them any information they will look for the odd pattern. In the real world this sort of thing could go on for a while before anyone noticed. But a good controller/facilitator can use this injection of information as a point of discussion during the design process. Would the system really react to this level of information? What level would it react to?

Since we don't quite know what the Virginia health system would react to, we have set out a limited number of cases. However, it is quite possible that on discussing the situation with public health and hospital personnel that they would not really alarm on a couple of cases of respiratory disease, even once it was diagnosed as Hanta. Sure, they would report it, and records would be kept, but the response system would not energize. If you figure this out during the design phase you can adjust the number of presentations so that the system is triggered, without being apocalyptic. If you wait and figure this out during play you will have to adjust dynamically. That is one advantage of having given them the numbers early in the day, before play really starts. If they shrug then control can easily go back and say, well, it's the morning of day 7 and look at all the additional cases you've been seeing! An experienced controller can do this and the players won't even be aware that the game scenario changed dynamically. They simply think the game was designed that way.

Turn 2

Now the rest of the cases should drop, with us going from Day 6/7 to Day 10. Setting the next turn to Day 10 picks up the rest of the cases. The first turn should have been focused on getting organized, communicating with hospitals, and waiting for confirmatory tests to come back. Turn 2 should be the next phase, where the response turns from a communication problem to an assessment problem. Players will need to assess what has happened, begin the tracing and investigation, and put together that this was a naturally occurring outbreak that happened at an overnight camp.

The key question is how they do this. What assets do they need, who provides them, and how the various organizations work together on the problem? There are also legal and medical requirements that need to be met, both with reporting and response. This turn will end with the players beginning to understand that this was a limited, naturally occurring, outbreak.

Turn 3

Turn three thus becomes a recovery turn, where the players have to build their communications plan and begin to notify and inform the leadership about what has happened. If possible, a mock press conference would be an ideal way of ending this turn. Bring in reporters from the local media, put them onto the control team, and give them a backgrounder on what has happened so far. The press will ask very realistic questions based on our experience, and give the personnel in the game a chance to see how their communications plan is working, and also a chance to gain experience talking to the media.

Chapter 17: Matrix Games for Disease Response

Matrix games are a technique that has caught on in the professional gaming community in recent years because:

- Matrix games can be short, with limited numbers of players
- These games have a formal structure that tends to support data collection
- This combination of short time span, limited numbers of players, and ease of data collection allows for games that explore topics that might otherwise not be explored in a game.
- They give the players, and the sponsors, a game experience, without the perception of all the work involved in building a large, complex, game.

There are challenges associated with matrix games, which make them particularly difficult for less experienced designers and controllers to pull off. This can create a trap of sorts, with the ease of the style luring inexperienced designers in, while they find the games surprisingly difficult during execution. Here we will briefly introduce the concept of matrix games and give references that cover the subject in greater detail. We will then focus on how to build matrix games for disease response, and some of the challenges and opportunities associated with doing so.

Matrix games

Matrix games are a form of gaming developed by Chris Engle as an extension of the role-playing format.[286] Matrix games come in many varieties, but the "classic" game has the following characteristics:

- *Between 5 and 11 players and a controller.* The players each represent something that has agency in the game. Players can represent a wide range of things, from the CDC to the President, to all left-handed Americans of Irish ancestry, to the weather. Generally, players represent organizations or individuals.

- *Each turn each player gets to assert one thing about the game.* It could be an action the player's role takes, or it could be anything about the game such as "it's raining." The key is that players get only one action, and the action cannot simply overturn another player's action. Think of it as improv theater—you have to accept other players actions once they have occurred, but you can then riff off of them.

- *Whether the stated action can occur depends on discussion among the players and ultimately on the assessment of the game controller.* Some actions – such as the CDC deploying epidemiologists – are inherent in the player's portfolio and simply occur. Others such as "I find the source of the disease" are subject to discussion and argument. The controller asks the player why they think their action will succeed and they give reasons (for example, "I deployed an epidemiological team, they are very experienced, and this disease is obvious). Other players may give negative reasons ("the lab is backed up, the family is uncooperative, and it takes time"). Using these various considerations, the controller may assign a probability to the action and roll a die to see if it succeeds or fails. Once an action has succeeded it becomes part of the game narrative and cannot be easily undone. But it can be modified by other player actions.

- *The goal is to have players engage in quick actions, adjudicate them quickly and move around the player group.* The more complex the actions, the more interrelated the player groups, and the more dependencies involved in actions the longer things can take. The game can take longer if there are also a lot of players, with the first player forgetting what they originally wanted to do by the time it gets back around to them.

The adjudication process can be simple or more complicated depending on the game design. Complex adjudication schemes include assigning an initial probability to the action's success and then modifying that probability according to player arguments. Different probability distributions can also be used. For some games "secret moves" provide additional complexity where players can engage in actions unknown to the other players.

---

[286] For a thorough introduction to matrix gaming see the following references: Curry, J., P. Perla, and C. Engle. (2018) *The Matrix Games Handbook.* Curry, J., T. Price, and P. Perla. *Matrix Games for Modern Wargaming.* (2017) Curry, J. and T. Price. (2014) *Matrix Games for Modern Wargaming: Vol. 2.* Curry, J. and T. Price. (2017) *Modern Crises Scenarios for Matrix Wargames.*

This, of course, defeats the nature of the game mechanic allowing players to debate whether and why an action succeeds. Generally secret moves are limited to one or two per player per game.

Matrix games are designed to build a shared narrative about a topic. Thus, whether a player "wins" or "loses" is less important than the way the player participates. Players and the controller are working together to evolve a narrative that provides insight about the topic. Because of the nature of the game, where only one player acts at a time and arguments are structured, it is also very easy to document a matrix game for later analysis.

Matrix games are deceptive, however. The player roles have to be structured so that each player has agency in the game – so that players can do and accomplish something. How the players are briefed on the game and their roles also matters for game play. Experienced hobby gamers work exceedingly well in matrix games, because they quickly realize how to use the structure to accomplish what they want. They work their goals into the overall narrative, building off other players actions, which increases their overall likelihood of success. Less experienced players can struggle to understand what they should do, and how to accomplish their goals.

The scenario for matrix games also matters a great deal. It has to direct and focus the action on the objectives of the game and has to be pitched at just the right amount and type of detail to stimulate the players to action. The scenario has to motivate players and give them the desire, reason, and ability to act in the situation, or the game will simply fizzle.

Finally controlling a matrix game is also more complicated than it looks. The controller has to ensure that each player makes a reasonable proposed action, but not allow players to engage in two actions during one move. They may also have to "fill in the blanks" to keep the narrative going or keep players in the game. Finally, they have to know how to manage game dynamics. If some players need to consult with each other prior to the turn (or should have done so but didn't) the controller needs to understand how to seamlessly handle the situation (e.g., ask the other player any predicate conditions assumed in the current player's move).

Matrix games are a useful tool that has developed considerable popularity in professional gaming circles. However, they have to be constructed with care and require an experienced, or at least confident, controller.

Matrix games for disease response

Matrix games work well for areas like research, evaluation of alternatives, and team brainstorming. In the case of disease response this would include activities such as:

- *Research.* This could range from research on disease epidemiology to new vaccines and treatment.

- *Behavioral health.* Many public health issues are related to the public's behavior. Vaping, for example, is a behavior that has health implications, but it is also associated with a complex range of political and policy issues.

- *Health management.* Deciding where resources go, or what actions an organization might take, can require consideration of a range of stakeholder inputs. If a hospital system were to consider opening a series of rural cardiology clinics only to find that the cardiology department thought they were unsupportable because of a lack of skilled nurses, that might be something to come out of a matrix game.

- *Policy issues.* Various departments have programs that they might be rolling out. Using a matrix game to understand the potential ramifications—legal, social, political, organizational, and health—for any new policy change might enable departmental leadership to identify potential problems before they occur.

- *National security games.* Here the disease is a challenge across the spectrum of government, and everyone involved needs to respond. This can be a strategic political game where each agency or government needs to formulate a policy, then decide what to do first.

- *Implementation of new technology.* As new technology is rolled out within a medical-care system the unanticipated consequences could be identified through a matrix game.

You will notice that in all of these examples we avoided tactical or operational disease response. That is because matrix games are not as well-suited toward on-scene response operations as they are organizational and policy discussions. While you can use them as a tool for these topics, the difficulties you will run into include:

- Time. A classical matrix game allows time to shift according to what players do in the game. In a tactical emergency response timing of the response governs player actions, not the other way around.

- Space. Most tactical emergency response games involve moving objects around and sending resources to various location. A classical matrix game has a hard time interacting with a map. Do players get free moves for everything on the map? If they do then their matrix moves focus on what, exactly? If they do not get free moves then their arguments about what is occurring on the map will either slow things down to a crawl or result in things that need to be simultaneous happening sequentially.

- Decisions. Player decisions in a matrix game focus on the arguments and how they convince others about their points. Decisions in a tactical emergency response are focused on the situation as much as the other players, and the dynamics of how the situation changes.

This does not mean you cannot use a matrix technique for these sorts of games. Only that it will be more difficult, likely require a great degree of abstraction, and confuse the players who are used to driving firetrucks around without having to argue about it.

Open ended problems without a fixed solution work better with the rigid and formal structure of matrix games than situations where multiple actions need to occur at the same time within the context of a plan or framework. In matrix games each player is identifying the most important task for that turn. This is fine if the players are experienced enough, and willing, to play along. That is often not the case.

For open-ended topics such as research on disease you can construct a matrix game where players represent a range of possible roles. For example, a matrix game on a treatment for a particular disease could include:

- Funders – government and non-government

- Companies – working the treatment for profit

- Academic and institutional researchers

- Regulators and reviewers

- The disease itself

In this game the companies, funders, and academics could reach whatever deals they wanted to in order to further research. Researchers and companies would argue their approaches and techniques, potentially divided into basic research, advanced research, product development, testing, and production. Each phase would need to be argued separately. Likewise, the regulators would argue about rules and data that would be needed. The discussion could become both detailed and technical if everyone in the room were an expert.

Including the disease as a player in the game may seem strange, but since we don't have a treatment, we likely don't know everything we need to about the disease. The disease player would be the player most experienced with researching the disease and would be able to give plausible extrapolations about the molecular biology of the disease as the game went along.

Recording the discussion would give insight into where and how progress might be made, and any challenges that might occur as different paths were taken.

Here the one action per turn limitation is an advantage, because it allows the group to stop and think about each proposed action and its implications for everyone else involved. The argument format will bring out both the advantages and challenges of a line of work. And the expertise of those experienced with the disease will be a powerful voice in examining different approaches. The controller will not necessarily need to be experienced with the disease, only familiar enough with the terminology and biological processes to be able to comprehend what players are saying.

The challenge with doing games involving response operations is that the players will often become confused or rebel. This is an important consideration for matrix games—they are highly stylized and game-like. Most seminar or tabletop games involve the controller facilitating any actions that the players want to take. Enforcing rigid structures onto players turns the situation into more of an actual game, which can go against both the players' common sense, and their desire not to be seen doing a "game."

Chapter 18: Pandemic Recovery Matrix Game

This is a matrix game designed to examine the interrelationship between the political, social, and medical decisions in a pandemic. It is not meant to project a specific pandemic as the focus is on some of the key challenges that could occur as a pandemic virus spreads, mutates, and challenges the ability of the system to adapt. This game was designed in the spring of 2020 with a direct reference to COVID-19. However, it quickly became out of date as the complexity and timelines for the COVID-19 pandemic changes.

This shows the difficulty in dealing with a current real-world event in a game. Things change, meaning the game design will need to be updated to account for the most recent situation and events. To avoid this, we dropped any reference to COVID-19 and changed the disease to COVID-XX so that we could build our own scenario independent from any real-world events, in order to have more lasting utility

Here we provide the basic components of the matrix game, components that can be adapted to the particular circumstances of the pandemic you want to simulate.

Background

In early October two years ago[287] one of many viruses being monitored by the Wuhan Institute for Virology changed as it jumped from one species of bat to pangolins.[288] From pangolins it jumped to a few human hunters and was circulating in the rural population of Guangxi Province. In October of this year the disease had mutated and adapted to its human hosts. Thus, when a well-known group of pangolin providers visited the Wuhan Wholesale Market[289] to sell their pangolin, two of the individuals traveling with the group were infected with SARS-CoV-X or COVID-XX. Because of the cool, wet, environment within the market it was an ideal venue for the virus to spread.

By the beginning of November an unusual respiratory illness was beginning to present at several clinics around Wuhan. By mid-November the virus had been referred to the Wuhan Institute for Virology for typing and testing. Within another week scientists at the institute understood that they had a unique virus that was in the SARS family and possibly spreading within the human population. Initial confusion about transmission delayed any major response until mid-December, at which point it was established that the virus was transmissible. By early January China had alerted international health authorities that a novel SARS Coronavirus was transmitting from humans to humans.[290]

At that point chaos and misjudgment took over. The Chinese Government took only marginal protective efforts; travel from Wuhan continued unrestricted until February. During that initial period there were only minor outbreaks in Asia, the US and Europe. By the time everyone realized a pandemic was upon them, it was March, and at that point serious protective measures—such as a lockdown of all non-essential activity— were ordered in several nations.

Current situation

In late March the US went on lockdown. Movement was restricted and non-essential businesses were closed. They are just beginning to re-open, but this varies with the business area and state. The economy has taken a significant hit with unemployment standing at 20%, high volatility in the stock market, and substantial losses to the travel, tourism, hospitality, and airline sectors.

What we now know about the virus is described in the SARS-CoV-X section, below. The lockdown in the United States continued through June, with increasing economic agitation to get the country re-opened again. In some countries, Korea and Japan for example, extreme social distancing and general compliance with public

---

[287] Relative dates are your friend. Because I'm using relative dates I am not tied to any particular year, but the wording is familiar enough for players to assume that it was last year.

[288] Pangolins are scaly anteaters, quite cute, and threatened by poaching.

[289] It's always a good idea to avoid direct references to actual activities in game materials, particularly when you are saying something bad about them. Unless it's a terrorist, in which case the reward you'll get from capturing a terrorist bringing a libel suit in federal court will outweigh the lawyer fees. The original market name was the Hunan Seafood Wholesale Market.

[290] If this sounds like the COVID-19 timeline that is because it is. No sense in re-inventing anything.

health instructions saw new cases of the virus reduced to almost zero. Other, more geographically isolated, countries such as New Zealand and Iceland saw the virus almost disappear. US political leaders have vacillated between reopening in the early fall and continuing restrictions going into winter.

It's now July.

Public health professionals are emphasizing social distancing, masks, and avoiding large gatherings where many people could become infected simultaneously. Their strategy remains to avoid overloading the health care system. They know that in the absence of an effective vaccine the number of cases, and corresponding fatalities, will reach herd immunity proportions under most foreseeable circumstances.

Several important policy decisions have not yet been made, and they remain on the table.

- How fast and far should reopening go?

- Should particularly vulnerable groups be segmented for isolation, like those over 65, while others remain free to work, associate in public, and enjoy themselves?

- What will the economic fallout be of self-isolation amongst a large segment of consumers?

    o In fact, the wealthy are spending far less than other segments during the lockdown, and even after limited reopening. If this continues the economic impact may be substantial amongst lower-wage service workers.[291]

- What should the government policy be if those who survived previous infection lose their immunity after a certain amount of time? Even more serious, once a vaccination is successfully created and distribute, what if that immunity is similarly temporary?

- The disease, and the disease response, has become increasingly politicized. In particular:

    o Conservatives and liberals view protective measures differently.

    o A militant anti-vaccination movement has emerged, along with several other alternative theories about the origin of the disease[292].

    o A divide has emerged between business and investment interests seeking to minimize the overall financial cost, and to get the economy working, and the labor and social justice movement that seeks extended unemployment benefits and other compensation for displaced workers.

    o Russia and China have both been tied to information actions on the Internet and elsewhere designed to exacerbate tensions and potentially delay economic recovery for the US. This includes manipulation of markets for supplies as well as competitive actions regarding vaccine research and production.

In some areas of the country the number of new cases of the disease has fallen consistently for the past two weeks. This, however, appears to be random with the exception of New York (state and city) and New Jersey. While rural areas were spared early on, there is now a substantial increase in cases in some rural areas, while others remain with few cases. California, Florida, Michigan, and Illinois all have seen substantial increases in the caseload, with no obvious cause other than people beginning to intermingle with greater frequency and in greater numbers than before the lockdown occurred in March.

This has led to a patchwork of recommendations, regulations, and timetables with each state and often local communities setting their own criteria for reopening.

Internationally those areas hit hardest saw their case numbers fall substantially, at least until they began to reopen. Now both China and Italy are seeing spikes in case numbers, causing at least China to impose significant movement restrictions in some provinces.

---

[291] Emily Badger and Alicia Parlapiano . "The Rich Cut Their Spending. That Has Hurt All the Workers Who Count on It" *New York Times.* 17 Jul 2020.. https://nyti.ms/2N5KilY

[292] Theories include it is an engineered disease by multi nationals to make money selling the vaccine, it is caused by 5G phone masts, and it does not exist.

As the country moves into the fall there is growing apprehension that the disease is not under control, preventative measure are failing, the disease has become a political issue, and US adversaries are exploiting this as an opportunity to further weaken the US as an international leader.

A couple of things everyone in the US needs to know:

- The Congress has passed, and the President signed, several trillion-dollar relief bills. Reimbursement for medical costs, unemployment insurance, and other relief measures were included in these bills. Some believe an even bigger program is needed, while others are sad that the original money was spent.

- As part of the series of large spending bills Congress has set limits for out-of-pocket medical expenses related to SARS. Beyond that limit the US government will step in and reimburse for medical expenses related to SARS. This legislation expires in August. Beyond August it will need to be renewed. Already there are arguments breaking out about the overall cost of writing a blank healthcare check from the federal government.

SARS-CoV-X[293]

SARS-CoV-X is a highly contagious Coronavirus with a low to medium mortality rate. While it is primarily transferred by droplets or nano-particles emitted during breathing or coughing, it can also survive on surfaces up to three days. The progression of the disease varies widely, and why that is the case is the subject of much research. What is known is that for those under 60 years of age there is only a slight chance (< 5%) of requiring hospitalization upon catching the disease. Between 20 and 40% of those catching the disease in this age group exhibit no symptoms, with between 10 and 20% of those remaining both asymptomatic and highly contagious.

The disease lasts for approximately 14 days with a range from 7 to 30 days and potentially even longer. For those that do become ill the most common symptoms are fever, trouble breathing, and aches and pains. Of those that do show symptoms 20% require hospitalization. Of these 10% require intubation with a 50% fatality rate of those receiving intubation. The overall fatality rate of the disease is between 1 and 2% of those who become ill, with the fatality rate rising to 15 to 20% for those over 60. The fatality rate increases even more for those over 80, with a 50% fatality rate if symptoms appear.

Younger people do present with the disease, with approximately 10% of those presenting with symptoms requiring hospitalization. Symptoms can vary widely in younger patients and range from cardiac problems, to renal failure, to a gastro-intestinal variant of the disease. One hypothesis currently being examined is that there is a wide variability in the strains of the disease, with some catching a mild strain while others catch a more virulent version of the disease. Recent studies in China are indicating that the disease has a high mutation rate in humans, resulting in approximately 50 variant strains being detected.

If the high mutation rate is true then antibody immunity may be difficult to achieve as the disease will change over time. This has been recently confirmed in studies of people who have come down with the disease more than once,[294] and in DNA typing of viral strains from China. This suggests that immunity to the disease is unlikely and individuals who have had the disease remain at risk.

Currently vaccine trials are occurring in several countries, with development and production of the vaccine receiving high priority. However, the recent studies coming out of China caution against optimism for a vaccine. Trials of a powerful steroid have shown some positive outcomes for the sickest patients in preventing the cytokine storm[295] which often signals that the patient is terminal. At minimum it is believed that aggressive steroid therapy will prevent some of the organ damage seen in severely ill patients, especially younger ones.

---

[293] Cutoff for references on SARS-CoV-2 is 23 Jun 2020. I am giving references for CoV-2 here in order to illustrate how to ground your fictional scenario in reality, and to ensure that I'm not creating something well beyond the bounds of what is possible. It also shows that the medical literature is often both a moving target and annoyingly contradictory and vague about the kind of details we need for games. But SARS-CoV-X is entirely fictional and should not be conflated with SARS-CoV-2.

[294] Long, Q., Tang, X., Shi, Q. *et al.* Clinical and immunological assessment of asymptomatic SARS-CoV-2 infections. *Nat Med* (2020). https://doi.org/10.1038/s41591-020-0965-6

[295] They hyperactivation of the immune system which can be life threatening. See, for example, Fajgenbaum, David C and Carl H. June. "Cytokine Storm," *N Engl J Med.* 383 2020 2255-2273.

Rules

This is a standard Matrix Game and is designed for one player to occupy each position in the game.

Play proceeds as follows:

- *Situation update.* If the controller has additional information or injects for the players, they describe them along with that moves starting situation.

- *Negotiations and planning.* Players get some time to talk to each other and think through their next moves in the game. Players may choose to do anything that is within the scope of their role's abilities. Any actions requiring coordination should be coordinated prior to the resolution phase.[296]

- *Player actions.* The controller goes around the table and asks players in turn what their actions are. The controller can decide what order to get the players actions in. The moves are not written down beforehand, allowing the players to adjust their actions according to other player's decisions. This will require some discernment on the part of the game controller who will need to decide if the player's reactive action is reasonable in the context of the game.

- *Resolution.* Player actions are resolved by the controller using arguments made by the moving player, and any supporting or counter arguments made by the other players. To resolve the action the controller sets a probability that the action will succeed and modifies it according to the arguments for and against success. Some actions will occur automatically, since they involve no one but the acting player, while others will be dependent on other players who must first agree. Once an action has been resolved it become part of the history of the game.

This is a very free and open form of game with a lot of responsibility placed on the controller. A more rigid scheme might involve players submitting written moves, and then a set of rules or guidelines to allow for some deviation from the moves depending on other player actions. This would also be a more closed format, with the possibility of players conducting secret moves.

Player roles

Matrix games should have no more than 6-12 player roles in order to speed things along. Obviously if you have a larger group, or a more complicated topic, you can have more roles in the game but then the game will take longer, and you will get through fewer turns. Here we include 10 roles in order to illustrate the variety of roles that you can have in a matrix game.

Player roles in the game are:

- White House
- Congress (both houses)
- Governors
- Business
- Department of Homeland Security
- Department of Health and Human Services
- Centers for Disease Control and Food and Drug Administration
- Public – the general public
- Testing and vaccines
- The disease

---

[296] I cannot emphasize this point enough. In a matrix game the resolution phase should be focused on player actions and their resolution, not ongoing negotiations between players. The most that the controller should need to do is verify that a player agreed to some other players actions if agreement is required. If you don't point this out to players, loudly and continually, they will not come to the resolution phase having had all the discussion they need, and the game will bog down. Note that this does not imply that coordinated actions automatically succeed, just that the players should do coordination prior to resolution.

If we want to reduce the number of player roles, say to six, then there are several options. First, we could begin by eliminating those roles with "less to do" which would be Health and Human Services and the General public. We would combine the CDC and HHS roles into one role (called HHS) and combined the general public and disease roles into one player – a joint public/disease player.

This would have the advantage of combining roles, like HHS, that have primarily an administrative and communications role with the operational role of the CDC. Likewise, the disease player may not wish to "activate" every round, so that player would alternate between being the "public" and the "disease." This is an example where the flexibility of matrix games can allow you to cover more topics and issues that a normal game with a limited number of roles.

If had a lot of players, but only wanted eight or ten roles, then you could have committees of players play some or all of the roles. This would allow player groups to discuss their actions prior to making a move, which increases player engagement. It also slows the overall game down, because players will need time to talk within their teams.

For each of the ten roles above we give a description of the role along with some background as to what they know that no one else does, along with what their motivations might be.

White House Briefing

You will need to decide which political party you represent at the beginning of the game and note it down (Republican or Democrat).

Reopening is picking up steam at just the wrong time. Or the right time. Depending on who you are. As more and more states begin to lift their lockdowns, allowing economic activity to resume, the number of cases in the US is going up. More worrisome is that cases are also going up internationally in countries that were "ahead" of the US.

And you have been given more bad news. The mutation rate of the virus may result in any vaccine effort's being futile. It may also mean that people who have had it once may get it again, and they may get an even more virulent strain than they did last time. The virus does not seem to be getting weaker, only stronger. This is not a good situation.

It's not good for two reasons. First it means that even with herd immunity at least some fraction of the population may always be susceptible to the disease. With a fatality rate of 1-2% that is 10 to 20 times higher than the fatality rate from seasonal flu. That's a lot of potentially very sick, or very dead, people going forward. This has two implications that are what is worrying you:

- If a substantial fraction of the population requires intensive care on a routine basis, the overall cost of health care will skyrocket. Already some insurance companies and hospitals are indicating that without government reimbursement they will have to either stop covering SARS, stop providing treatment, or go out of the health insurance business.

- While businesses are reopening, consumer confidence remains mixed. In particular the wealthiest 5% of the population, who account for a large fraction of service and discretionary spending, have significantly pulled back on spending. This is because higher net worth individuals primarily spend on services and travel, both of which are difficult to consume in the pandemic. These individuals can also afford to leave crowded cities, and work from remote destinations. If this continues, or gets worse, then the country will likely fall into a deep recession or even depression. The demographics that are currently spending, the lower middle and middle classes, do not have enough money at the end of the month to really move the economic needle.

- Internationally you are concerned that China and Russia will take advantage of the situation. The whole problem of who gets the vaccine first, and what they will do with it, is of great concern because it could be highly destabilizing.

You need to restore consumer confidence, fix the health care system, and find a way out of this disease. Should be easy, you are the President.

Congress Briefing[297]

You represent both houses of Congress, and both parties. While the Republican's do not have a majority in the House, they do have a slim majority in the Senate. Thus, if anything is going to get done the Republicans will have to agree to it. This opens up an enormous range of possible actions for you. If any money is spent you have to agree to it. If you suspect something is wrong you can investigate it, possibly decreasing the overall political capital of the White House. You can, in fact, investigate as both the Republicans and Democrats during subsequent turns.

You will need to consider the situation carefully, as it can be difficult to get things done in a divided government. What are the political consequences for both parties if something is approved or voted down by the Congress? What is likely to pass? You set the criteria and the agenda, keeping in mind some of the real-world trade-offs involved.

Governors Briefing[298]

You represent all of the governors in the US. You can decide to be the governor of California one turn, and the Governor of Alabama the next. Or you can represent all of the Governors and describe the overall situation. You could close the whole country or open it. And the federal government cannot do a lot other than try and persuade you.

You are concerned that if you don't open up you will be criticized by businesses, if you do you will be blamed for the next outbreak. How much risk are you willing to take? How much will the government support you?

Business Briefing

You represent the business community within the US. This includes the financial, manufacturing, transportation, agricultural (industrial), and medical sectors. You also represent the small business community. As institutions that depend on both production and demand you would like to see things open up as quickly as possible. However, this is tempered by your economic models that show if you have too much disease the economy will suffer both through productivity loss as well as self-isolating decisions, and if you open too late you will damage the ability of businesses to restart.

The medical community you represent has the same issues, they want to reopen because many of the elective and routine procedures that have been put on hold are the ones that actually pay the bills. With SARS they are losing money despite being full.

You are predicting that the economy, both big and small industries, could be crippled if things don't get restarted. And the problem is both being physically open, and also that consumer demand comes back online. Consumers, particularly the wealthier ones who have significantly curtailed spending, need to be confident enough to make major purchases. The entertainment and travel industries are particularly concerned about this.

---

[297] Given the current divide in the US's politics it is not possible to have a "bipartisan" Congress. However, in games players frequently disregard their titles and work together in wholly unrealistic ways. While in recent years this has begun to change with more acceptance of the divide, you can't control player actions to that degree of detail.

[298] This is your "out" if you have a large group and need additional player positions. There are 50 US States each with a Governor. Just remember – time goes up with each player added!

Department of Homeland Security Briefing

You are the overall coordinator for the non-medical portion of the response. HHS is in charge of medical issues. Where, exactly, one set of responsibilities ends and the others begins is not well defined, but you tend to focus on hardware and support, while HHS focuses on medical and medical infrastructure.

One thing you are in charge of is the supply chain. Or not, depending on how you want to play it. Passing off the supply chain to others risks loss of coordination and lack of efficiency, but it also means that you have fewer things to play for, worry about, or get blamed for. This means:

- Acquiring test kits, especially PCR probes once they are approved by the CDC and licensed by the FDA

  o You would have to manage all of the infrastructure surrounding delivery and distribution

- PPE for hospitals and others

  o There is no national inventory or distribution system so right now its everyone for themselves. Ventilators have the same problem.

- Food and other essentials

  o It is possible that the overall supply chain for essential materials will get disrupted. It has already begun to fail in Mexico.

  o If this happens it will be much harder for you to dodge responsibility but how will you mobilize capabilities to support the system if key nodes like harvesting or processing or distribution go down? You don't have a spare cold-storage warehouse capable of feeding the New York City area.

You are also in charge of constructing emergency facilities like hospitals (and possibly morgues) if things get bad enough. The Department of Defense can help with this; however, they are very expensive.

Health and Human Services (HHS) Briefing

You are the focus of the response – and are coordinating across your various departments (NIH, CDC, FDA, SAMSHA). It has not been easy; each department tends to want to go its own way and hold press conferences about it. This has not made the White House happy.

You are now in a situation where individual's mental health has begun to be affected by the lockdown. SAMSHA is working to support mental health issues but needs a significant plus-up, and some sort of legislation to ensure that mental health is covered both through the SARS special legislation (coving expenses related to SARS) as well as through private health insurance. Violence has been rising and SAMSHA clinicians believe this may be due to both the virus as well as the lockdown.

Lockdown related violence has been primarily domestic, while virus-related events seem to have both a viral and a frustration component associated with them.

Of course, you are also working on a vaccine, treatments, trying to manage hospital capacity, all the while trying to make sure everything is done in a reasonably safe and secure fashion.

Your biggest concern is that you don't understand this disease very well, and something else could happen to make things worse.

SARS-CoV-X cases have continued to decline in US metropolitan areas over the past several weeks. Both imposed and self-isolation has led to a manageable, but crushing, number of cases showing up at hospitals. The primary areas that have been affected so far are urban areas. But now rural areas are beginning to see spikes as well, but at lower levels than urban areas.

Models show that removing lockdown will eventually return the level of disease to its pre-lockdown trajectory. Until either herd immunity (60-80% immunity) or a vaccine is developed, any remains of the disease will eventually grow into a major event.

Asymptomatic but infectious spread is one of the primary means of spreading the disease, which is why testing, and isolation of positive tests is the only way to really contain the disease. The current testing regimes suggest that no matter how strict the isolation imposed there will be a remnant of the disease which can re-infect the population.

Your biggest problem is that *The Lancet* will publish a peer-reviewed, well thought of, article tomorrow that strongly suggests immunity for the virus will last 2-6 months with an average of 3.5 months. The mechanism for this loss of immunity is the genetic variance of the virus—there are currently 50 identified strains—and its relatively high mutation rate. This article is based on genetic analysis of current outbreaks in China amongst populations already thought to be free of the virus. The article will also indicate that there are long-term, persistent, factors for the disease, both in terms of organ damage as well as re-emergence of the disease. It is possible the disease could re-emerge in a patient who tested antigen-free six months or more after they had the disease.[299]

The one *silver lining* is that the variance in immunity seems wide; some show immunity even after months, while others infected in May have already lost immunity. Right now, the maximum observed period for immunity is 6 months. Figuring this variance problem out is critical to vaccine development.

Testing is a brain puzzle. There are two types of tests. One for the antigen – do you have the disease, and one for the antibody – have you had the disease and/or been vaccinated so you are "immune." You have several good tests for each, however, for both types of tests, and all the tests selected, there is a significant false positive/false negative rate. Looking at it as a matrix, table 6 shows what the problem is.

Prediction	True Condition		
	Positive	Negative	
Positive	True positive (TP)	False positive (FP)	Total positive rate
Negative	False negative (FN)	True negative (TN)	Total negative rate
	Recall = TP/(TP+FN)	Accuracy = (TP+TN)/Total	Precision = TP/(TP+FP)

Table 6: Confusion matrix[300]

In the tests that you are rolling out the both the false positive, and more importantly, the false negative rates are too high. This means that you are missing a lot of potentially asymptomatic but infectious people in your test. No one fully realizes the potential flaws in the false negative rates of the tests, primarily because of the asymptomatic nature of many individuals and the current chaos at the laboratories. It is likely that the

---

[299] This is a noteworthy change from SARS-CoV-19 which is thought to have at least partial immunity provided by having the disease, and that vaccines will work. This disease will essentially have no herd immunity, will be more like the common cold, and will keep attacking with it 2% fatality rate for virtually forever. This will pose a significant challenge to the players. You can obviously modify it, but such a challenge will mean they will have to go down certain paths, such as communications and prevention, that they would not otherwise go down.

[300] The accuracy reflects how well our test is doing amongst all of the tests taken. Recall is the fraction of all possible positives that we have successfully predicted. And precision is the fraction of all the positives that we got right. See, for example, https://towardsdatascience.com/decoding-the-confusion-matrix-bb4801decbb

overwhelming number of samples arriving at the laboratories as you roll out the kits is partially responsible, but another likely cause is ineffective use of the kits by untrained workers giving the tests.

There have also been studies in recent days showing that there are individuals with very low levels of virus in their blood, and who are also asymptomatic. These individuals appear to still be capable of spreading the virus but may be at levels below the detectable limit for current testing. This may represent 10-20% of all symptomatic cases.

Players in games don't always have to represent organizations. To demonstrate that we are going to put in a few wild-card player roles. These player roles will work best in matrix games where they will create the conditions for the other players. But they are also useful in standard seminar games where subject matter experts or others can be assigned these roles in order for them to bring their experience to the table.

As the testing player you are the actual tests. There are a lot of them, from different manufacturers and using different techniques. You determine the overall effectiveness of the tests – some tests may be more intrusive than others (finger pricks vs nasal swabs) and that may affect the overall reliability of the tests.

There are three general types of test: antigen (do you have it), antibody (have you had it) and environmental (is this spot contaminated). Right now, there is a high false positive/false negative rate on all the tests. False negative rates are bad because it allows someone who could potentially be infectious walk around spreading the disease. It is possible that some individuals have lower antigen levels than can be detected by the current crop of tests, which means that even a really good test won't detect them.

You need more money for tests and can assert that unless you get it (from FDA/Congress) that the tests aren't working. You could also say that the approval process has been rushed, and the tests aren't working. Or you can claim that a manufacturer has falsified numbers.

You can also decide to roll a die on the testing table, which you can use (or threaten to use) if you run out of arguments. You can also simply select results from table 7 regarding success/failure or production numbers and give them to the other players.[301]

D10	Antigen	Antibody	Environmental
1	Fails FDA testing/6 month delay (-2)	Fails FDA testing/6 month delay	Does not work at all
2	Reengineer 2 month delay (-1)	Too many false positives 3 month delay	Does not work at all
3	Reengineer 1 month delay (-1)	Too many false negatives 2 month delay	Does not work at all
4	Reengineer 1 month delay	Production problems 2 month delay	Production delayed 4 months
5	Production problems 2 week delay	Production problems 1 month delay	Production delayed 2 months
6	Start immediate production	Start immediate production	Start production immediately
7	1000/week production	100,000/week	Start production immediately
8	10,000/week production (+1)	500,000/week	10/week production
9	100,000/week production (+1)	1 million/week	100/week production
10	1 million/week production (+2)	10 million/week	1000/week production

Table 7: Testing player results table

---

[301] This represents a very "free" type of game where players and controllers get a lot of leeway in how they approach their roles. In a more ridged game, the testing table might be consulted every turn to see where things stand with testing and the results simply applied as a condition of the environment.

And, yes, it is possible to put the tests into production (many already are) but then find out that the tests need re-engineering.

You also control the outcomes and actions regarding vaccination. If anyone tries to develop a vaccine you can make arguments about timelines, dosages, political considerations, and effectiveness. One thing to consider is the duration of any immunity involved in the vaccine.

Public Briefing

You represent the public in the game. All of them. You can be panicked, shocked, irritated, or just plain stubborn. All at the same time. You get a vote (literally and figuratively) on how the other players are doing, how the response goes, and when you go back to your normal lives (unless the government players impose mandatory lockdown in which case you can cause civil unrest if you desire to). In order to accommodate this vast power, you have the following special abilities:[302]

- You have an ability to interrupt another player and claim that the public will reverse whatever decision the player is making. You need to make an argument and the argument needs to be successful (according to whatever rules you are playing by). This interrupt is evaluated separately from whatever action the player is taking (obviously if the player can't take the action their move ends).

- You determine White House and Congressional poll numbers.

- You determine what actions other countries, and other interests, are taking to upset and manipulate the situation.

You don't represent any one group or fraction: you represent all of them. One turn you may be focused on antivaxxers who are totally against all forms of vaccination and testing, while on another turn you may be those concerned with the social justice aspects of the government's response. Or you could be both on the same turn.

You don't represent businesses, but you do represent customers. You decide whether customers are going back, going out, and complying with rules and regulations. If you favor the business player you could be responsibly consuming with social distancing and PPE, or you could favor the disease player and go out partying with no masks or distancing. You can also strike (think food service workers and teachers), lobby Congress, or crush someone at the polls.

Each turn you should consider the following:

- Public willingness to participate in business operations (purchasing, travel, entertainment)

- Employee sentiment and willingness to show up in person and accept a return to normal compensation.

- The poll numbers for the administration and Congress.

- The willingness of the public to participate in disease mitigation actions like testing or vaccination.

You can negotiate with players, extort them, or punish and reward them.

Examples of some of the things you can get irritated about:

- Medical workers are short on PPE due to supply chain issues or corruption

- Food supply becomes spotty due to disruptions in the agricultural system

- Grocery store and restaurant workers refuse to show up

- Businesses are not paying enough or providing medical benefits

- Unemployed individuals are starting to get very upset as the benefits approved by Congress expire and they begin to lose health insurance and any prospects for a job.

---

[302] From a design perspective these abilities are important because, just like with the testing player, other players can ignore the views of the public and just proceed with whatever they wanted to do in the first place. This, of course, happens, but there are usually consequences for elected officials. These rules try and put that pressure on the other players. And they give the public player agency in the game that they might not otherwise have. This is an example of where rigid rules can help a free form game along in special circumstances.

Public Sentiment

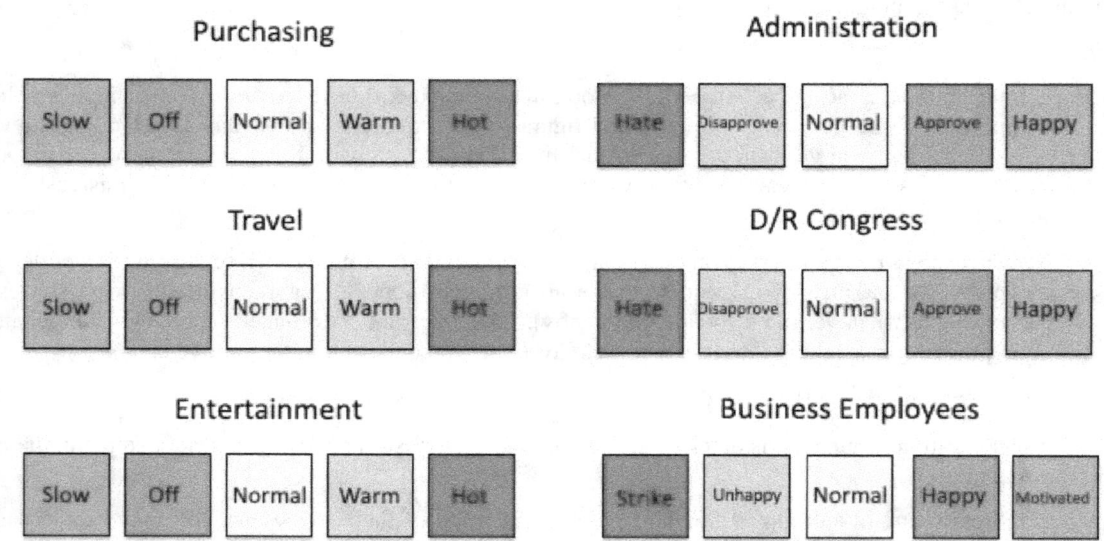

Figure 7: Public sentiment track- Using colors helps players visualize the situation. Slow is blue, off is green, normal is yellow, orange is warm and red it hot

You can use the track in figure 7 to keep track of public sentiment.

Disease Briefing: SARS-CoV-X

You are the disease. As such you have some decisions to make. What is your future in this world? How will you evolve? Your goal is to infect as many people as possible, and to stay around as long as possible. Look at the common cold – it's the most successful virus in history. Your goal is to match or equal that, at least until all the hosts run out.

The way you accomplish this goal is through mutation. You can change your transmissibility, lethality, and mutation rate, but be careful – if you become too deadly you can end up burning out quickly. If you spend your time mutating you may also make a mistake and allow for herd immunity, die out, or lose your sweet asymptomatic spreaders.

Each turn you may do the following:

- Provide descriptions of effects and outcomes. So, for example, if you have a large outbreak in a rural state, say Nebraska, you can assert that the health system in Nebraska is overwhelmed, many don't live close enough to take advantage of the system anyway, and that many are dying alone and unobserved on their ranches and farms. This should have some effect on the public player. You can also claim various locations, such as military bases or businesses are affected, or make other claims about the virus.

- Choose 3 or fewer areas of the US to increase (or decrease) the case load in. You can adjust the numbers in up to 3 geographic areas (states, cities, regions). The smaller the area, the wider the swing can be. You can specify any medically related fact in your description. For example: "there is a major outbreak in Houston and the hospitals are overwhelmed, in fact mortuary services are overwhelmed and they are looking to refrigerated warehouses to house the dead."

- Increase or decrease your mutation rate one square. The mutation rate will affect lethality and transmissibility, but you will need to roll on the transmissibility and lethality tables in order to determine what the outcomes are. You can change your mutation rate and choose not to roll on the table that turn.

Disease display

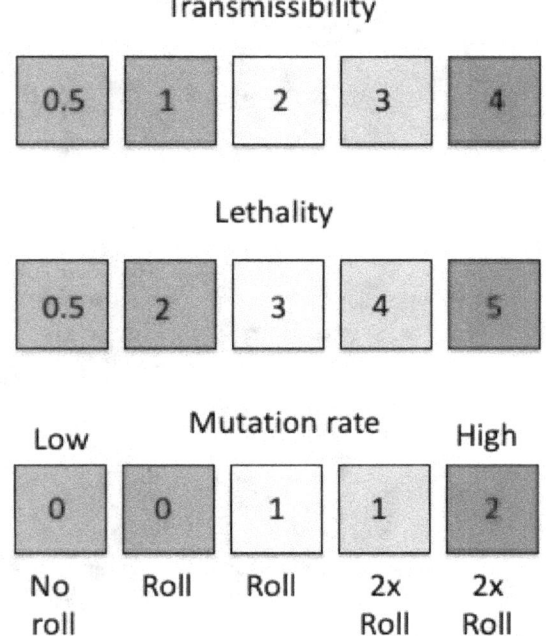

Figure 8: Disease display: No roll is blue, roll 0 is green, roll 1 is yellow, 1 2 x roll is orange, 2 2 x roll is red

The mutation rate table (figure 9) allows you to change your lethality, but at the risk that the epidemic gets under control. Each turn you choose whether you want to roll on it. You can only roll once per turn unless your mutation rate is orange or red. Then you can choose to roll twice if you want to (i.e., see the first roll, then decide whether you want to roll again). The mutation tables give you both the results for your die roll in terms of how the transmissibility (T) and lethality (L) move on the disease display (figure 8) but also the lethality and transmissibility give you your overall cases and fatalities in millions.

You can roll straight on the table, or you can use the mutation bag. If you use the mutation bag place 1 green (-2), 2 yellow (-1), three blue (0), 1 orange (+1), and 2 red (+2) tokens in a bag. Each time you roll on the table you pull a token out of the bag and apply the associated modifier to the die roll (D20). You will notice that as you pull more of one type out of the bag, your chances of having the opposite occur increase.

Disease mutation tables

Mutation roll (D20)

1: L and T +2
2: L+2 with no impact on T
3: T+2 with no impact on L
4: T and L +1
5: L+1
6: T+1
7-14: NE
15: L-1
16: T-1
17: T and L -1
18: T and L-2
20: Herd immunity

Roll on table, for each 1 on drift draw a high/low bonus cube from bag

Cases (million)

Lethality	Transmissibility				
	0.5	1	2	3	4
0.5	1.25	2.5	5	7.5	10
1.5	0.625	1.25	2.5	3.75	5
3	0.5	1	2	3	4
4	0.375	0.75	1.5	2.25	3
5	0.25	0.5	1	1.5	2

Fatalities (million)

Lethality	Transmissibility				
	0.5	1	2	3	4
0.5	0.025	0.05	0.1	0.15	0.2
2	0.0125	0.025	0.05	0.075	0.1
3	0.015	0.03	0.06	0.09	0.12
4	0.015	0.03	0.06	0.09	0.12
5	0.0125	0.025	0.05	0.075	0.1

Figure 9: Disease mutation table. Roll a D20, apply the results to figure 8 showing the transmissibility (T) and lethality (L) of the disease. Read the current cases and fatalities (millions) off the associated tables.

This table means that you have some choices to make. Roll on the table and things can get better for you (and worse for the other players) but they might also get worse for you. This mutation stuff is a dangerous game. You cannot simply change the disease at a whim, that would give you too much power over the other players and be unfair. However, one of the challenges with disease is that it is dynamic and can responds to host actions.[303]

Control

Control has the role of facilitator, as well as adjudicator and inject creator. The way the game should work is that the government takes actions, and the public, business, disease, and testing/vaccination players react to those decisions. The public, business, disease, and testing players are creating the scenario dynamically, feeding difficulties and challenges into the other player positions. As facilitator your primary job is to create and facilitate this feedback loop. Otherwise, the players will simply be looking at you to resolve all of their actions in terms of disease spread and outlook.

You should also consider the trade-offs for the disease carefully if you do not want the disease player to have the possibility to create either a super lethal, super contagious disease, or the opposite. Putting some boundaries on the disease's ability to argue for increased transmissibility or lethality would increase realism at the expense of taking away some regions of disease for the players to explore. And you should note to the disease player that they can make many other arguments other than transmissibility or lethality; for example, they could argue that a particular venue, like airplanes, are areas where the disease propagates more effectively than other places.

---

[303] https://www.scripps.edu/_files/pdfs/news-and-events/The%20D614G%20mutation%20in%20the%20SARS-CoV-2%20spike%20protein%20reduces%20S1.pdf

Execution

About one to seven days prior to the game beginning the players should be given the general scenario, and information about their roles. This will give them a chance to read the materials before they arrive at the game. Based on our experience about 20-30 percent of players will arrive having read the materials. Of the rest 10% will have read it over in great detail and have a lot of questions, and the remainder will not have read it at all. This applies to all games, not just matrix games.

The game should begin with an overview briefing of the game scenario and situation. Players should also be given a detailed explanation of game play, with emphasis on what constitutes a valid argument. Examples can help here, as can sample moves from the facilitator.

Because the game play is somewhat stylized, and because it all hinges on arguments made by the players, the facilitator should go over the process of adjudication in detail, using plenty of examples. One area to explain in great detail is the difference between what the facilitator will accept the player can do in one move, and what facilitator decides will require two moves. In our games we often define one move as having a consistent focus, while two moves will be about two different things. For example, a player wants to deliver vaccines from a stockpile to the affected area. This would normally involve removing vaccines from the stockpile, putting them on a plane, sending the plane, taking them off, inventorying them, and breaking them down for distribution to vaccination sites. This would be one move, because it is focused on vaccine delivery. If, however, the player wanted to vaccinate people at the location, but no vaccine had been delivered, then they couldn't include delivery along with vaccination because those are two different processes.

The facilitator should also emphasize that any agreements, negotiations, or other activities between players should be finished prior to the adjudication phase of the game, so that these actions don't delay the game. Ideally all the facilitator should need to do is simply confirm that the other players agree with the move, but often the players forget to mention to other players that they will need something from them for their move to succeed.

In this game it will be important to explain the role of the disease, public, and vaccine players both to the actual players in those roles as well as the rest of the players. These are not "normal" roles to play in a game and some orientation will be needed.

Play then proceeds through a series of phases each turn:

- Situation update. The Controller will provide an update on the situation, including a summary of the players' actions. This will baseline the world for that turn.

- Planning phase. Players should be given a chance to figure out what they want to do that turn, and to talk to other players. Placing a short time limit on this phase will be important as most players will take all the time available plus whatever extra time you give them.

- Player actions. This is where the facilitator goes around the table and resolves the player moves.

In the following sections we elaborate on each of these phases. Game play will continue until the objective have been met, the players have run out of ideas, or time runs out. The facilitator should reserve a half-hour at the end of the game for a hot washup discussion of what was learned and why the players made the decisions they made.

Situation update

At the beginning of each turn you provide the players with any additional information you want to give them as the facilitator. This opportunity can be used to expand on player actions or limit the overall effects of a player move. For example, if the disease player decides that the overall lethality of the disease is increasing – then you can say that is not the result of a mutation but rather a finding based on additional epidemiological data and only seems to pertain to congregant living facilities, especially prisons. This represents a control inject, but it has the effect of elaborating on the player move, expanding the problem set for the government players (now they have to address prison populations) and giving the public player some ideas (like riots in prisons). This makes you as much a player in the game as the other participants, but your role is slightly different. Your role in describing the initial situation is to:

- Make sure the players understand the current situation. For example: "We have had outbreaks last turn in the Midwest that have significantly increased hospitalizations and taxed hospital capacity. The public is facing long-term high unemployment and has begun looking to Congress to act on a relief bill. The airlines have claimed they are going out of business in another three turns unless their needs are met for financial relief."

- Adjust, expand on, and elaborate player moves. The example above is one way to do this. You can also simply point out to the players what other players have done last turn, so that they are aware of the situation.

- Help the players think through their next moves. As a controller you should have a bigger perspective than the players and are more familiar with the material. You can make connections between player moves, for example: "The Congress just passed a mandatory mask law, if I were the public (looking at the public player) I might have a reaction to that…"

In larger, seminar games, or tabletop games these "scene setters" are often done as pre-prepared "injects" that control inserts into the game. Since virtually all aspects of reality are represented by a player in this game, control's role is more complex than would usually be the case in a facilitated game.

The key is to maintain game play and player interest, help players who are either less knowledgeable or experienced, and maintain the game's general direction toward the game objectives.

Negotiations and planning

As the facilitator you should give the players enough time to think about their moves and talk to each other. The White House will likely want to provide policy and guidance to HHS and DHS and consult with the Congressional player. The Congressional player may want to talk to the public and business.

At the same time, you should insist that if the players need to coordinate about something, they should do it during this phase instead of waiting to the resolution phase. There is nothing more time wasting or aggravating in a matrix game than to have the players start negotiating a move in the middle of resolution. The most that should be needed is for you to ask the other players who need to agree to a move whether they agree. If they do not then that is something for the players to resolve the next turn.

How long should this phase be? It should be long enough that the players can get their discussions done, but not so long that they feel free to negotiate at length. The players should feel pressure to prioritize and get their work done quickly.

Player actions

Once the players are finished negotiating you go around the table, each player describes their action, and you work with the players to resolve the action to your satisfaction. There are a couple of decisions that you have:

- *Player move order.* You decide who goes when. You can either do this as the game goes along or establish a set order. Remember that players can change their moves after hearing other player's moves so move order can matter. The players with the most options, and the most authority, in a situation would generally go last. Or the player with the initiative, the one driving the situation at that point, could go first and set the agenda for all the other players. Typically, this might be the disease, public, testing, and business players. The then other players react to what they are doing.

- *One move only.* Players will frequently attempt more than one move per turn. This can be incidental, deploying a vaccine will require many individual actions to occur, or deliberate, attempting to do two different things at the same time, say react to moves by both the Business and the Public. The latter is an obvious violation of the "one move per turn" rule, but the former, where multiple actions add up to one action, is not. You will need to decide whether an action is a single action or multiple actions. One way to do this is by deciding whether the actions are related and supporting one, common, goal. Another is whether the actions are above or below the "level" of resolution in the game. If the game is at the strategic level, worrying about national policy, then the sequence of manufacture of vaccines is below the level of resolution of the game.

- *Resolving arguments.* Many player actions are obvious and will succeed unless extraordinary circumstances occur. The CDC deploys epidemiologists. That does not require a success or fail roll. On the other hand, if a player takes an action that may or may not succeed you can open the resolution up for discussion. Players will give reasons why the action would succeed or fail, with a limit on one to three reasons per player. You decide whether the arguments are worth considering, and how much they affect the overall outcome. You can simply decide or roll a die against a probability of success you have established. When adjudicating, it is better to favor arguments and actions that are clever, unexpected, and build off of other player actions. That keeps the game interesting, and interactive. It also encourages creative play on the part of the players. The bias for any adjudication should be toward success. However, success is not always fully successful, and can have parts that backfire. So, failure can mean that the action happens, but creates more challenges for the player. So, for example, a player claims that the new vaccine they have developed turns out to be 95% effective. The adjudication is that is true, but only for one particular strain of the disease. Or that some parts of the population have negative reactions to the vaccine, pregnant women, for example.

As each player's action is completed and resolved you will note down the result. This builds a narrative for the game and is a very important element of running a matrix game. Especially if you are forgetful. With 10 players making 10 moves per turn that are interconnected and shape the world, after 3 turns that means you will need to remember 30 things unless you write them down. I find it helpful to have someone assisting with the role of transcribing moves and keeping track of what is going on. They can back you up in case something relevant happened a couple of turns ago that you forgot about.

The game proceeds around the table until the objectives for the game are met, the players run out of steam, or time is called.

Bibliography

Alibek, K (2000) *Biohazard: The Chilling True Story of the Largest Covert Biological Weapons Program in the World.*

Brauer, F. et al. (eds.) (2008) *Mathematical Epidemiology.*

Caffrey, Matthew. (Jan 2019) *On Wargaming.* Newport Papers 43. https://digital-commons.usnwc.edu/newport-papers/43/

Caves, J. and S. Carus. (2014) *The Future of Weapons of Mass Destruction: Their Nature and Role in 2030.*

Carus, S. (2001) *Bioterrorism and Biocrimes: The Illicit Use of Biological Arms in the 20th Century.* https://wmdcenter.ndu.edu/Publications/Publication-View/Article/626562/bioterrorism-and-biocrimes-the-illicit-use-of-biological-arms-in-the-20th-centu/

Celentano, David and Moyses Szklo. (2019) *Gordis Epidemiology, 6th Ed.* Elsevier. 2019.

Center for Counterproliferation Research (National Defense University). (Nov 2002) *Anthrax In America: A Chronology and Analysis of the Fall 2001 Attacks.* https://wmdcenter.ndu.edu/Publications/Publication-View/Article/626576/anthrax-in-america-a-chronology-and-analysis-of-the-fall-2001-anthrax-attacks/

Centers for Disease Control and Prevention. Recent Incidents https://emergency.cdc.gov/recentincidents/

Centers for Disease Control and Prevention list of bioweapons https://emergency.cdc.gov/agent/agentlist-category.asp

Curry, J., P. Perla, and C. Engle. (2018) *The Matrix Games Handbook.*

Curry, J., T. Price, and P. Perla. *Matrix Games for Modern Wargaming.* (2017)

Curry, J. and T. Price. (2014) Matrix *Games for Modern Wargaming: Vol. 2.*

Curry, J. and T. Price. (2017) *Modern Crises Scenarios for Matrix Wargames.*

Ellis, Devin. (2020) "'Crimson Contagion' – What can we learn?" *PAXSims Blog.* https://paxsims.wordpress.com/2020/03/19/crimson-contagion-what-can-we-learn/

Fenner F. et al. (1988) *Smallpox and its Eradication.*

Gursky, Elin, Thomas Inglesby, and Tara O'Toole. (2003) "Anthrax 2001: Observations on the medical and public health response." *Biosecurity and Bioterrorism: Biodefense Strategy*, Practice, and Science. 1:2.

Howard, Andrea (1 May 2020) "The Pandemic and America's Response to Future Bioweapons," *War on the Rocks Blog.* https://warontherocks.com/2020/05/the-pandemic-and-americas-response-to-future-bioweapons/

Johns Hopkins University, Red Cross, and Red Crescent. (2007) *Public Health Guide in Emergencies 2nd Ed.*

Ketheesan, N. (ed.) (2012) Melioidosis*: A Century of Observation and Research.*

King R. and Curry J. (ed) (2015) *It Could Happen Tomorrow! Emergency Planning Exercises for the Health Service and Business.*

Leitenberg, M. et al. (2012) *The Soviet Biological Weapons Program.*

Martcheva, M. (2010) *An Introduction to Mathematical Epidemiology.*

Purkitt, H. and S. Burgess (2005) *South Africa's Weapons of Mass Destruction.*

Perla, Peter with John Curry (ed.). (Aug 2012) Peter Perla's *The Art of Wargaming*, 2nd Ed.

Saffer, B. (2004) *Anthrax (Diseases and Disorders).*

Sanger, David, et al. (22 Mar 2020) "Before the Outbreak a cascade of warnings went unheeded." New York Times. https://nyti.ms/2U1tyAs

Steward, Antony. (2002) *Basic Statistics and Epidemiology.*

Timbrell, John A. (2009) Principles *of Biochemical* Toxicology, 4th Ed.

United States Army Medical Research Institute for Infectious Diseases. (Sep 2014) *Medical Management of Biological Casualties (Blue Book) 8th Edition.* https://www.usamriid.army.mil/education/instruct.htm